The Riding Doctor

The
Riding
Doctor

A Prescription for
Healthy, Balanced, Beautiful Riding
Now and for Years to Come

Beth Glosten, MD

RiderPilates® LLC

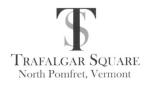

TRAFALGAR SQUARE
North Pomfret, Vermont

First published in 2014 by
Trafalgar Square Books
North Pomfret, Vermont 05053

Disclaimer of Liability

Exercise can be dangerous, especially if performed without proper pre-exercise evaluation, competent instruction, and personal supervision from a qualified fitness professional. Always consult your physician or health care professional before performing any new exercises or exercise techniques, particularly if you are pregnant, nursing, elderly, or if you have any chronic or recurring medical problems.

The techniques, ideas, and suggestions in this book are not intended as a substitute for medical advice. Any application of the techniques, ideas, and suggestions in this book is at the reader's sole discretion and risk. The editors, author, and/or publishers of this book make no warranty of any kind in regard to result from the information in this book. In addition, the editors, author, and/or publishers of this book are not liable or responsible to any person or entity for any errors contained in this book, or for any special, incidental, or consequential damage caused or alleged to be caused directly or indirectly by the information contained within.

Trafalgar Square Books and Beth Glosten encourage the use of approved safety helmets in all equestrian sports and activities.

Note: The "Rider's Challenge" stories in this book are works of fiction. Although the author has based the stories on her clients' actual experiences, the names, places, and incidents are the product of the author's imagination. Any resemblance to actual persons, living or dead, events, or locales is entirely coincidental. The stories titled "My Challenge" are true and depict the author's personal experiences.

Library of Congress Cataloging-in-Publication Data
Glosten, Beth.
  The riding doctor : a prescription for healthy, balanced, beautiful riding, now and for years to come / Beth Glosten, MD.
    pages cm
  Includes bibliographical references and index.
  ISBN 978-1-57076-664-0
  1. Horsemanship--Health aspects. 2. Exercise--Health aspects. 3. Physical fitness. I. Title.
  RC1220.H67G58 2014
  616.89'16581--dc23
                      2013047190

Illustrations by Sandy Johnson
Photographs by Audrey Guidi (all exercises); Carolynn Bunch (pp. 3, 4, 7, 18, 20, 42, 47, 56 *bottom,* 61, 64, 75, 83, 89, 100, 106, 112, 117, 123, 127, 129, 139, 147, 152, 156, 168, 170, 173, 177, 178, 184, 186, 191, 197, 199), and Tim O'Neal (pp. 16, 48, 56 *top,* 62, 125, 150, 155, 158); Cindy Cooke (p. 1); Doug Hartley (p. 21); Cappy Jackson from *The Rider's Guide to Real Collection* by Lynn Palm and used by permission (pp. 28, 132, 175); Beth Glosten (pp. 53, 55, 59, 63, 67, 190).
Book design by Lauryl Eddlemon
Cover design by RM Didier
Typefaces: Minion, Roboto Slab

Printed in China

10 9 8 7 6 5 4 3 2 1

Dedication

This book is for committed riders of all skill levels and disciplines looking for ways to understand and improve themselves for better performance and health.

Contents

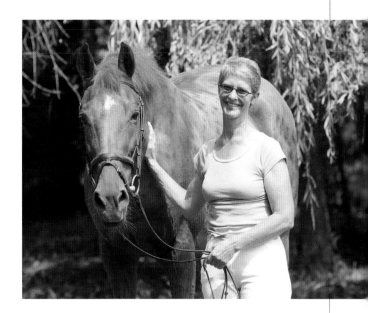

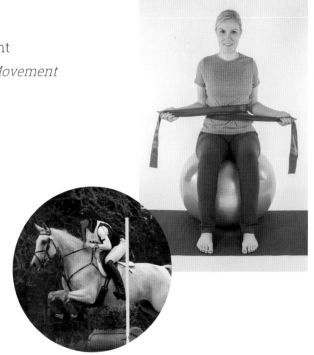

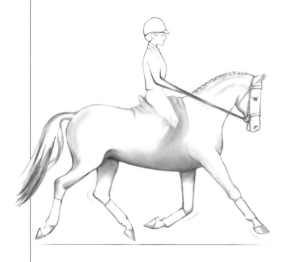

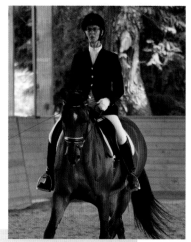

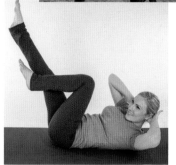

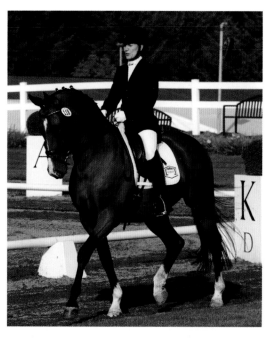

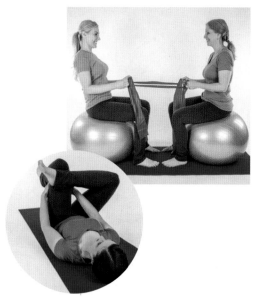

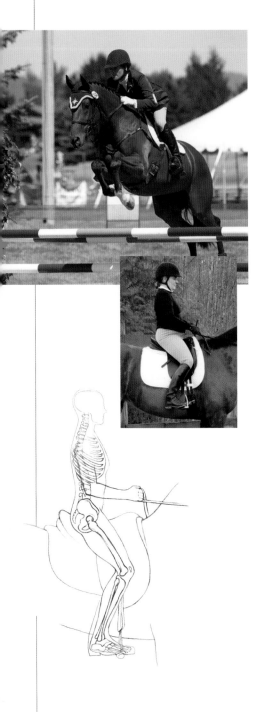

Acknowledgments

I am grateful to my many wonderful, thoughtful clients who asked questions that helped me clarify my ideas and urged me to forge ahead with this project. I also thank my beloved equine partners—my most important teachers.

I am very grateful for the expert drawing skills of Sandy Johnson. Thank you Bonnie Snow, Carol Miller, Mary Cox, and Courtney Secour for being models for the exercise photographs. Thank you Audrey Guidi for taking the time away from two young daughters to photograph the exercises. Thank you to Carolynn Bunch (Carolynn Bunch Photography) and Tim O'Neal (Action Taken) for their expert horse and rider photographs, and thank you to the riders willing to appear in the book. I am grateful to Dr. Andrew J. Cole (Executive Director, Musculoskeletal Services, Swedish Health Services; and Medical Director, Swedish Medical Group) for reviewing parts of the book.

It was a great pleasure to work with Publisher Caroline Robbins and Senior Editor Rebecca Didier at Trafalgar Square. I so appreciate their enthusiasm for the project and guidance to its end.

Glossary of Terms

You'll find the following terms in the pages ahead—here's a quick primer:

Abduction. Movement of a body part *away* from the center of the body.

Adduction. Movement of a body part *toward* the center of the body.

Anterior. Facing *toward* or located in the *front*.

ASIS (Anterior Superior Iliac Spine). The prominent part of your pelvis just below your waist, sometimes referred to as your hip bone.

Balance. A state of bodily equilibrium. Balance is a condition of stability produced by even distribution of weight on each side of a vertical axis.

Bones. Form the rigid structure of the human skeleton. Bones are the levers that muscles move. Bones are connected with ligaments across joints.

Dorsiflexion. Decreasing the angle of your ankle joint. When standing, lifting your toes off the floor dorsiflexes your ankle.

Eversion. Refers to the ankle joint and involves both abduction and dorsiflexion and results in the bottom of the foot facing away from the center of the body.

Extension. In general, a movement at a joint that increases joint angle. From the anatomical position (standing, forward facing, arms by your sides, palms facing forward), extension of a limb brings it behind you. Therefore, extension of your spine results in *bending backward*, and extension of your hip joint brings your leg behind your body. An exception to this terminology is the ankle joint: extension of the ankle, or pointing the toe, is called *plantar flexion* (flexion of the ankle is called *dorsiflexion*).

Flexion. In general, a movement at a joint that *decreases* joint angle. From the anatomical position (standing, forward facing, arms by your sides, palms facing forward), flexing a limb brings it in front of you. Therefore, spine flexion results in *bending forward*, and flexion of your hip joint brings your leg in front of your body. The exception is the knee: flexion of your knee, while it decreases joint angle, moves your lower leg behind you.

Focus. Keen attention to the job at hand.

Harmony. Cooperation and good communication. This is accomplished on horseback when you have good balance and aid timing so your horse can clearly hear you. Proper training of your horse assures that he responds to the aids. Good communication is then possible.

Inversion. Refers to the ankle joint; involves both adduction and plantar flexion (pointing your toes) and results in the bottom of the foot facing toward the center of the body.

Joint. Links bones together. Some joint configurations include a hinge joint (elbow joint and knee joint), and ball-and-socket joint (hip joint and shoulder joint). Joints are made of fibrous connective tissue and cartilage, and are supported by ligaments.

Loin. Some texts make reference to the rider's loins. Wikipedia defines this body part as the side of the human body between ribs and pelvis, or refers in general to the area below the ribs, or the general lower part of the body. This word has also been used to refer to genitals (hence the derivation of the term loincloth). Loin is not an anatomical term used in medicine, so I do not use it in this book.

Muscle. The contractile elements that move bones in relationship to each other. Muscles act by getting shorter and pulling—muscles do not push. The movement of bones in many directions results from muscles pulling in different directions. Muscles connect to bones via tendons.

Neutral Spine Alignment. Alignment of the spine such that its normal curves are present. When lying supine, *neutral pelvic alignment* is defined by the pubic bone and right and left ASIS being in a plane parallel to the floor.

Posterior. Facing *toward* or located in the *back*.

Posture. Alignment of the spine.

Relaxation. Mental or physical lack of tension. Relaxation is not a word I apply to riding. The mental component is not a trait I recommend while riding—a rider should be paying attention! Focus is a better word. Physical muscle relaxation is not what we seek while riding, but rather a cooperative tone that supports a stable position in motion. The word "relaxation" is often used when *balance* and *suppleness* would be more suitable. Muscle efficiency and organization, not relaxation, creates beautiful and graceful movement.

Rotation. Movement of the body in a horizontal plane. Rotation is either *internal* (*toward* the center of the body) or *external* (*away* from the center of the body).

Self-Carriage. Responsible for one's own balance. For the rider, this means not relying on the reins for balance, and staying steady with the horse without gripping with the legs.

Supple. Just the right amount of muscle tone and effort at the right time, resulting in fluid and controlled movement. Supple movement is graceful movement.

Tension. Mental or physical lack of relaxation. Appropriate tension is needed to support upright posture on the moving horse. This tension should not be restrictive, but rather a coordinated muscle effort that creates stability.

Riding in Balance

I am a medical doctor and I ride dressage. Hence, I call myself a "riding doctor." I wear this label when I work with riders and evaluate their balance and functional challenges on horseback. I do not diagnose medical disorders, but I use my background in medicine, movement, and riding to identify postural and muscle imbalances that can preclude effective riding, and cause or contribute to injury.

Riding in balance with a correct position creates the wonderful picture of horse and rider moving as one. I strongly believe that this position is not a gift conferred to just a few. *You,* too, can learn to ride this way. The journey starts by understanding a bit about how your body is put together and how to access the tools within yourself to support balance and suppleness. Not only will you improve your riding skills, but you will also be doing yourself a favor.

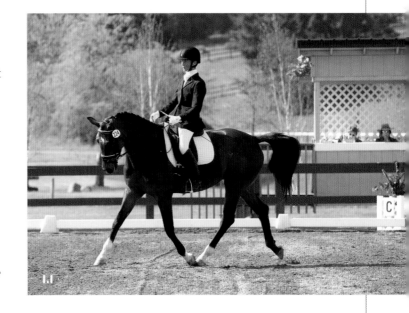

Here I am riding my 2004 Oldenburg mare Donner Girl ("DG") at Training Level in 2010. It is my hope that she and I can have a longstanding partnership and progress together through the levels of dressage. To do so requires that I take care of her, and myself.

The tools for graceful riding are the same ones we all need to ride in a healthy way: Correct posture and spine alignment creates not only a beautiful position on horseback but also the healthiest position for your body—one that promotes balance and efficient use of your many joints, minimizing unnecessary wear and tear.

My goal with this book is to empower you to understand your body and use it as effectively as possible while riding (or doing any other activity) so you are able to continue for years. But with the challenges of equestrian sport comes the requirement that you take care of yourself. Pay attention to your body. Use it mindfully, efficiently, and effectively. Ride in balance and ride in good health (fig. I.1).

My Story

I was fortunate as a teenager to have my own horse to love, ride, and care for. I enjoyed hours of riding bareback on the beach, jumping every log I could find on the trail, and growing up in the Pony Club system of rider education. Then, like many, I left riding for a number of years. After college, medical school, and residency training, it was time to have horses in my life again. What a challenge! Not only was it a struggle to balance my academic medicine career with my avocation, riding was really hard. Gone was the natural balance I had as a 12-year-old. Also gone was the complete lack of fear and the steadfast confidence that my horse could not unseat me. I struggled with tension and awkwardness. My back ached after I rode.

My frustration with riding prompted me to put on my "medical hat" and apply my clinical research skills to figure out what creates a harmonious "pretty picture" of horse and rider moving together. A firm believer that knowledge is empowering, I rode with different instructors and clinicians, reread anatomy books, and spent hours analyzing my own riding and that of others—whether proficient or not. I came to some conclusions:

First, learning—or relearning—to ride (or any other physical ability) in middle age is much more challenging than learning to ride as a preteen. As you get older, it is more difficult to learn new motor skills. It takes time, patience, and awareness to overcome ingrained movement habits that interfere with stability, balance, and symmetry. It is not impossible, however, but you need determination and a plan.

Second, I saw that many riders lacked some basic (but not easy) skills of core stability, and shoulder- and leg-muscle control. The rider who looks "one with the horse" moves in the right places—usually subtly at the shoulder girdle and arms and particularly at the hip joints—and is stable where necessary, in the trunk or torso (I use these terms interchangeably) of the body. A balanced rider is so in several aspects: balanced thought, that is, suitable focus without unnecessary stress; balanced spine alignment in correct posture; balanced use of the muscles of the shoulder girdle to accomplish elastic and steady contact; balanced use of the muscles of the hip joint for leg control as well as support to give the horse an aid at the correct time. A great rider's apparent ease comes from this controlled use of the body.

My study of rider function became more urgent when I ran into back problems. While back pain had plagued me on and off for much of my life, in my late thirties, it screamed at me with herniated lumbar discs. I tried everything to make life comfortable, but in the end, surgeries were necessary to take care of the problem.

I knew that in order to keep riding I needed to place renewed focus on fitness. I religiously did my physical therapy exercises and experimented with different exercise programs. The Pilates system of exercise was my portal into the body awareness I needed in order to improve my posture and change harmful movement habits (fig. I.2). I was fortunate to have patient and perceptive teachers who got me out of the "just do it" model of exercising, and guided me to focus on *how* I did an exercise.

DG and I in 2013. DG is a now a bit older and better balanced. I'm a bit older, as well. I work hard to preserve my posture, and hence balance, despite the effects of age. Mindful exercise, as described in this book, has been extremely helpful.

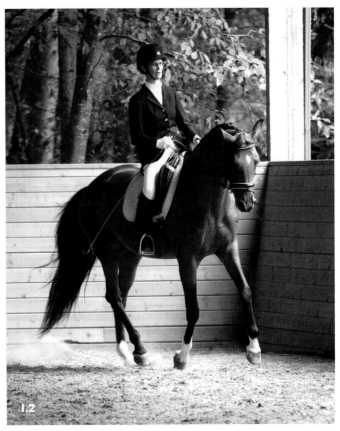

I.2

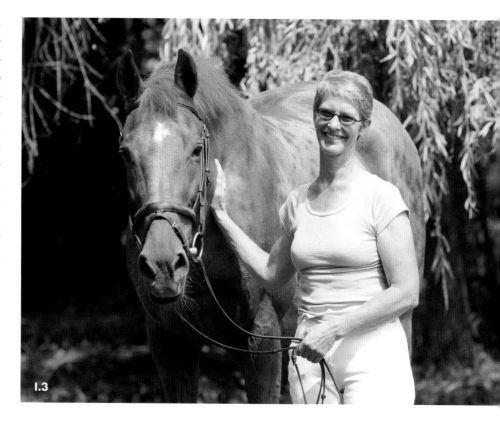

I enjoy some time at home with Bluette, my semi-retired 1992 Danish Warmblood Grand Prix mare. What an amazing journey I enjoyed with this horse: She was my first horse after my back surgeries. She was my partner as I learned the advanced dressage movements, and we competed successfully at the FEI levels, including Grand Prix. This horse has a huge place in my heart. I wish for everyone this special bond with an equine partner.

1.3

This opened up a whole new dimension of thinking about riding. While fitness is necessary, good riding goes beyond how much weight you can lift or how many sit-ups you can do. Good riding comes from fitness combined with body awareness, respect, and control.

I am a student of posture. Not only is correct posture crucial to minimizing further damage to my back (both while riding and going through life), it is also the basis of a good position in the saddle. I am continually amazed at how small positive changes in posture can markedly improve a rider's sense of security and balance, as well as the horse's way of going. Good posture is good for your back health and good for your riding!

I am now retired from the practice of medicine, and my second career is teaching my own RiderPilates® program that includes off-horse exercise classes as well as position-focused riding lessons. I continue to ride dressage and am diligent about maintaining my fitness. I have been fortunate to have some wonderful horses over the years, and since my back surgeries, I've ridden successfully at Grand Prix and have earned my USDF gold, silver, and bronze medals (fig. I.3).

I've worked with hundreds of riders in dressage and other riding disciplines, from rank beginners to experienced trainers. In both the studio and in riding lessons, I focus on posture and spine alignment, and independent and balanced function of the shoulder girdle, and the muscles of the hip joint and leg. I assess muscle imbalances and alignment issues that add up to dysfunctional balance strategies and inefficiency in the saddle, some of which cause pain. My goal is for you to organize your ride mostly from the center of your body (core), with the rein and leg aids added in. I believe the horse can "hear" the intent of your center—more forward, less forward, for example. Riding from your core improves the clarity of your aids.

I've found notable postural issues in over 90 percent of the riders I've worked with. Some issues may be subtle: For example, a small change in the balance of the pelvis in an experienced rider improves freedom and expression in a canter pirouette. Other postural issues contribute to harmful and painful misalignments of the spine and threaten your balance; insecure balance causes compensatory tension and dysfunction in the muscles of the shoulder girdle and hip joint, risking joint irritation and pain, and poor balance also increases the risk of a fall. Finally, inefficient balance and poor posture can disrupt the horse to such an extent that his gaits become irregular.

Beautiful riding is not magic. The skills for balanced riding can be learned and harmful movement and riding habits replaced with those that are more productive, not only in terms of training your horse, but also in taking care of yourself. Develop these tools off the horse to spare your horse from enduring your struggles with imperfect symmetry and coordination. Riding is a very busy environment; by improving balance and posture off the horse and focusing just on yourself, you can return to the saddle with a more organized body.

This book presents my system of rider evaluation and correction in what I hope you'll find to be a systematic, easy-to-follow way to identify and address your posture and balance issues. The body awareness and skills taught in the off-horse exercises will equip you with the needed tools to improve your riding.

By helping you understand how your body interfaces with your horse, I hope to help you meet your riding goals and, at the same time, ride in good health and prevent injury.

My approach is based on anatomy and how the human body works. I present the skills you need to ride well and offer specific exercises to teach these skills.

The Five Rider Fundamentals

This book is organized into five chapters, with each chapter focusing on one of the Rider Fundamentals (see list below). Each chapter includes a discussion of the relevant anatomy, and exercises are presented that teach the skills of the Fundamental. In addition, common rider problems and rider's stories clarify the relevance of the Fundamental to riding.

This list of Rider Fundamentals was inspired by the Dressage Training Scale for horses, which sets priorities and goals for training. I think it makes sense to have a Training Scale for the rider, too. When I teach, I use these Fundamentals to prioritize and organize the issues I see in a student. Use this list to organize your body in the saddle and improve your riding skills—in parallel with training your horse.

The five Rider Fundamentals are:

1 Mental Focus: Consider every step of the ride in terms of you and your horse. Be constantly aware of your position, and how your horse is moving (p. 11).

2 Proper Posture: Stay in a correct posture and balance and maintain this position despite your horse's movement and the application of your aids (p. 23).

3 Body Control—Legs and…

4 Body Control—Arms: Control your legs and arms and you'll have truly independent aids. Your legs and arms can move with and communicate with your horse without upsetting your balance and position, and your aids can be given in a way that enhances, rather than interferes with, your horse's way of going (pp. 85 and 131).

5 Understanding Movement: Understand the rhythm and basic mechanics of each of your horse's gaits and translate that into a logical way of moving with your horse at each gait, with appropriately timed aids (p. 157).

The Rider Fundamentals outline the skills you need to be able to ride effectively and with empathy—using your body efficiently and not getting in your horse's way. This list is a useful "on-the-fly" tool to help sort out how you, the rider, could unknowingly be contributing to difficulties with your horse. For example, if you struggle riding a shoulder-in, ask yourself, "Am I focused on the movement? Am I in balance? Am I gripping against the movement? Am I in rhythm with my horse, giving appropriately timed aids?" With the Rider

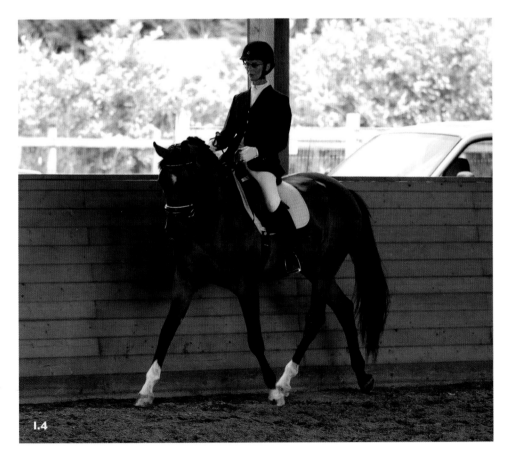

1.4

DG and I, in 2013, riding in left shoulder-in. The successful execution of lateral movements requires the rider to use all of the Rider Fundamentals: staying focused on the movement; proper spine alignment; coordinated body control of leg and rein aids; and moving with the horse. I'd like this photo better if I had been looking up more, and my upper back was less rounded.

Fundamentals, you can make sure you are doing your part to contribute to the successful execution of a movement or exercise (fig. I.4).

All these Rider Fundamentals are closely related and interdependent and should be developed at the same time. The Fundamentals will equip you to improve the precision and subtleness of your riding as you and your horse progress in training. For example, the novice rider can start by mastering all elements of the Fundamentals at the walk and begin to feel how she can move with the horse. On the other hand, the advanced rider will benefit from referring to these Fundamentals—the basics of good riding—when she is starting the four-year old prospect, or perfecting a Grand Prix jumper.

Overcoming Challenges

Throughout this book, in stories titled "My Challenge," you'll read more about my personal riding struggles and how I solved them. In "The Rider's Challenge" stories, you'll find fictionalized accounts of my real students' riding and health issues and how we worked together to improve their riding effectiveness—and enjoyment.

Exercises

The exercises in this book, some of which are adapted from the Pilates exercise system, can be done on their own or added into your current fitness program. They require very basic equipment, and my instructions focus on how to do the movement for maximum benefit. These exercises are not just about getting stronger: They are about learning where you are and how your body parts move. They are about improving your awareness of your body's foibles and asymmetries, then finding the tools within your body to override these lifelong bad habits—habits that show up dramatically in the precarious environment of riding. You can find a complete list of the exercises in this book on p. 201. Whenever an exercise is named in the pages ahead, you can locate it easily by referring to the complete list.

Of note: The models shown doing the exercises are not fitness instructors but are dedicated clients of mine who have stuck with this program to improve their health and riding.

Simple Exercise Equipment

You will need these inexpensive items:

Exercise Ball. There are many types and brands of exercise balls available. I have even found some for sale at my local organic grocery store! Purchase a ball that, when fully inflated, enables you to sit with your hip and knee joints level, or with your hip joints slightly higher than your knee joints (fig. I.5). You should neither feel as if you are sitting precariously high nor feel you are sitting too low in an easy chair. I have found that a 65-centimeter ball is a good size for the majority of adults. You can adjust the ball's inflation to fit you.

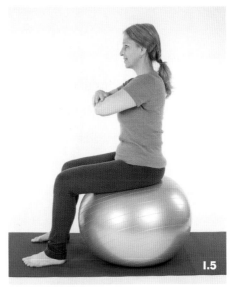

The correct exercise ball size: When seated, your thighbone should be parallel to the floor, with your hip joints level with, or slightly above, the level of your knees.

Mat. Almost any kind of mat will do: The goal is for you to feel comfortable lying on your back or on your stomach on the floor. For some, a towel on top of a carpet is enough.

Weights. I usually start out with 2 pounds. For some this might be a bit heavy, especially if you have had a shoulder injury. If you choose a heavier weight, pay very close attention to how you do the exercise so as not to hurt yourself. Never make the exercise so difficult that you can no longer pay attention to form and posture. Start small.

Stretch Bands. I use elastic stretch bands for many of the exercises in this book, and for the Partner Exercises in chapter 4 (see pp. 138 and 140). These bands come in a variety of strengths and degrees of resistance. I use a band of moderate resistance. (For all of the leg stretches, however, a large towel that allows you to hold both ends will suffice.)

More Nuts and Bolts

Before you start a different exercise program, check with your health care provider. I have done my best to provide a written description of the exercises to make them clear—and safe. However, without feedback from a trained instructor, it can be challenging to do them correctly. So, if any exercise causes you pain, stop; that shouldn't happen. Skip that one, and seek feedback from a qualified instructor before trying it again. My mantra for exercise is, "Mindful, careful, patient, progressive," *not* "No pain, no gain!"

I place great emphasis on the rider's role in the success of the horse-rider pair. By paying attention to her position and balance, the rider is equipped with the tools necessary to direct and manage the horse's energy and balance. Although I have ridden to Grand Prix, and I certainly recognize the horse has his own issues with body control and function, I will not be addressing these in this book.

What's more, although I'm a licensed physician I do not give medical advice—diagnose or offer treatments—in this book. My goal is to give guidance about rider position and function that I think is logical considering how the human body is put together. These same anatomy considerations apply to riders that struggle with pain while they ride. I have learned a great deal about the anatomy and function of the human body from various educational pursuits (medical school, Pilates, my own injury and rehab programs), but I am not a physiatrist, rehab doctor, orthopedist, or physical therapist. My medical background (and the academic side, for sure) equipped me with analytical tools that help me sort out rider issues. It has inspired what I hope you find to be a straightforward presentation of rider function in clear language that is understandable and consistent with human anatomy and movement.

Some of my ideas about how you can best use your body in the saddle are different from those voiced by other authors and riding experts. I believe that this underscores the challenge of using words to describe how to move, especially when there is the complication of another moving animal involved—your horse!

1 Mental Focus

The first Fundamental, *Mental Focus*, is the foundation for all of the others. Mental Focus means that you come to your ride prepared to fulfill your role as your horse's leader and are prepared to commit positive and unwavering attention to the job at hand. It means that you recognize the importance of—and practice—continuous awareness of your body position and your horse's movement. In this chapter, I'll look at the value of Mental Focus and give you some exercises to help you tune in to your body and stay present every step of your ride.

The skill of Mental Focus will also maximize the benefit of all of the exercises in this book. Use your awareness to feel your body during the movements. Embrace the purpose of the exercises and carry the connections they confer in your body into the saddle. Extensive skills of posture and body control get lost if they are not on your mind when you ride! Your riding will benefit when you constantly consider the organization of your body; you will better perceive how your horse moves and can make subtle corrections to his way of going.

Your horse requires you to be his leader—I like to call this role "benevolent alpha," that is, you are clearly in charge, and do so in a nice way and a clear way. This optimizes training. Without a commitment to your leadership role it is impossible to communicate clearly with your horse. At best, your vague aids result in a dull horse, disinterested and unaffected by your unfocused attempt

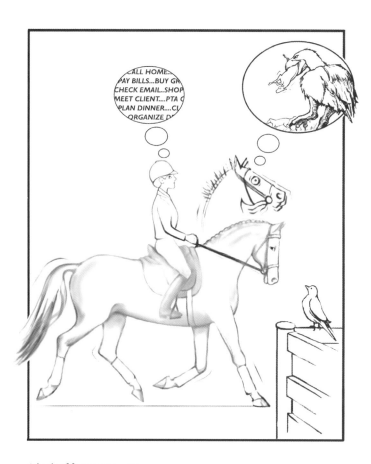

A lack of focus on every step of the ride leads to an unfocused and distracted horse.

at communication. At worst, you fall into an unhealthy posture and repeat ineffective and unbalanced riding habits, or your horse, sensing the lack of a clear leader, becomes dangerous and spooky, taking over and concerning himself with distractions and events unrelated to you or the ride.

Finding a clear mindset is not always easy. Work stresses, family needs, and other responsibilities conspire to divide your attention during a ride. When you settle in the saddle, you owe it to your horse and yourself to quiet the chatter in your head and commit all your energy to the ride. From this place you can fill the role of a guide who assesses every step. For this purpose, I have developed the 10-minute pre-ride set of exercises listed at the end of the book (p. 203). I designed this short series of simple exercises to get you out of your *head* and into your *body* before you sit in the saddle. These set you up for positive focus on your body position and function, and how you interface and interact with your horse.

Coordinate Your Breathing with Movement

On those days when stress makes it difficult to focus, take some time to settle before you get on your horse. Review your breathing once you are in the saddle (see the *Rib Cage Breathing* exercises beginning on p. 14). This breathing helps you to get out of your busy, noisy head and into your body. It helps to reduce tension in your shoulders and puts positive energy in your torso to support your balance and posture. When you lose focus during a ride, let this breathing bring you back to your body and your horse's movement. If this fails to shift you into a good riding mindset, make a note of it. Don't "flog" yourself; either reduce expectations or go for a trail ride!

Coordinating your breathing with movement promotes mental focus on any physical activity, whether your exercise workout, work around the house, or riding. When stressed for time, or in the electric and tense environment of a horse show, this breathing technique helps me to slow down and make sure my mind and body are on the same task: It is balancing, organizing, settling and it prepares me for the next exercise or movement. Because of my previous back injury, I use it before I get in my car or lift a bag of groceries, my horse's saddle onto her back, or a bucket of water. The preparatory and organizing feature of this breathing is why I call it the "rider's half-halt" (I use the same technique when riding a half-halt on the horse).

Rib cage breathing is active, balancing, and energizing. It involves a *lateral* and *outward* expansion of the *rib cage* while breathing in (inhaling), and a drawing in of the deep abdominal muscles toward a stable spine while breathing out (exhaling). It is the *exhalation* phase of the breathing that promotes balance and support, as it activates and directs your focus to the deep muscles of your lower abdomen and back so they are "on" and ready to support you during movement. Directing the inhale breath to the rib cage allows you to keep this core muscle support while you inhale.

This makes rib cage breathing different from the relaxing "belly breathing," which involves a release of the abdominal wall as you breathe in. Breathing into the rib cage, rather than releasing your abdominal muscles, allows core muscle support to be maintained during inhalation. In "belly breathing," the relaxation of your core muscles with the inhale breath reduces support of your body and is therefore less suitable during activity.

Rib Cage Breathing 1

Learn rib cage breathing while you are lying on the floor. This position helps you feel whether or not the bones of your spine move while you breathe. The alignment of your spine should not change.

1 Lie on your back on a mat or towel, knees bent, feet flat on the floor hip-joint width apart.

2 Take in a normal breath. As you exhale, let your rib cage drop slightly toward the pelvis, and gently and carefully pull in your abdominal muscles. This movement should feel fluid, not braced (this takes practice). Place your hands on your lower abdomen to feel that the muscles scoop inward. Avoid pressing your abdominal muscles outward, causing a braced feeling in your lower abdomen. This inward movement of the abdominal muscles should not move bones: Your lower back should not press into the floor. Your rib cage should not push off the floor. Your spine and pelvis bones should not move.

3 With each *inhale* breath, work to expand the lower, posterior part of your rib cage, but don't let your upper chest rise up. Keep your abdominals scooped in.

4 With each *exhale* breath, feel your focus and energy concentrate in the lower abdomen—in your center.

If you are having trouble keeping your abdominals scooped in as you breathe in, place your hands on the sides of your ribs. As you inhale, imagine your ribs swinging outward, or laterally, toward your hands. In fact, this is the way ribs are intended to move: like a bucket handle swinging out to the side as you breathe in. When done correctly, rib cage breathing should feel as if you are creating your own elastic corset of torso support. The engagement of your deep abdominal and back muscles should create a feeling of the rib cage and pelvis being elastically connected and knitted together.

Rib Cage Breathing 2

Having mastered rib cage breathing lying down, you'll now review it in a much more practical position—sitting upright!

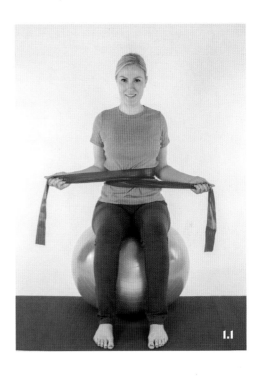

1 Sit upright in a chair or on an exercise ball, feet flat on the floor, hip-joint width apart. Align your body so that your shoulders are over your pelvis (see more on this in chapter 2).

2 Wrap a towel or a stretch resistance band around your midsection, cross it in front of your body, and hold one end in each hand (fig. 1.1). (If you don't have a stretch band, you can use your hands instead: Place one hand on your abdomen and one hand on your back.)

3 Take an easy breath in. As you exhale, gently pull on the ends of the band or towel so it squeezes around your middle. (Or, imagine your hand on your abdomen pressing toward your hand on your back.) As in *Rib Cage Breathing 1*, pull your abdominal muscles inward as you breathe out, and allow your ribs to drop down and in slightly (but don't round your body forward). It should feel as if you are making the space inside the towel or stretch band smaller.

4 As you breathe in again, keep muscle tone in your lower torso, expanding your ribs out to the side.

If you practice this breathing technique many times a day, it will gradually become more natural. Learning the breathing while sitting upright makes the exercise more relevant to riding. Begin each ride by taking a few breaths in the saddle to help you feel connected to the middle of your body.

Breathe when you are stressed and harried, and before you need to lift something. Practice in your car and use it to divert your mind from frustrating traffic: Breathe and center and take satisfaction that you are learning to organize your body and keep your brain quiet and focused. Soon it will become a positive habit of preparing and balancing your body.

A Pretty Picture

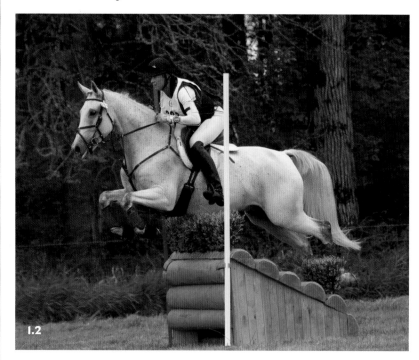

1.2

Karen O'Neal guides her 2006 Hanoverian/Shagya gelding Cowboy Casanova (aka "Hugo") over a very narrow cross-country fence. Here is an example of focus promoting safety. Karen notes that Hugo can be spooky and quick to duck to one side before a fence. While approaching this tricky jump, Karen must be very sure she is centered and on task. A rider who backs off of "riding every stride" while jumping risks poor preparation for a change in footing or a difficult approach to a fence. Things happen quickly at high speeds. Focus and pay attention!

RIDER'S CHALLENGE ||||||||||||||||||||||||||||||||||||||||||||||||||||||||||||||||||||||||||||||||||||||||||||

Lack of Focus

I arrive at Pines Farm as Rachel is warming up her 12-year-old Arab gelding, Mucho, in the arena. "I'm concerned about our lesson today," Rachel says, bringing Mucho to a walk. "The hay truck is supposed to arrive soon, and I'm sure he'll be upset and spooked by it."

Rachel looks nervously down the driveway. She cautiously moves Mucho back to the track in a posting trot, occasionally glancing at the road. Mucho, meanwhile, trots hastily with a hollow frame and pricked ears out to the environs. When he looks to the outside of the arena, Rachel snatches at the reins. Mucho hollows more and quickens his already tense trot.

"I hate it when Mucho is so distracted—it is just not fun," Rachel comments.

My challenge today is to help Rachel focus on the job at hand—riding. My goal is to quiet her active imagination and help her ride with a positive mindset to keep Mucho *with* her rather than passively waiting for him to spook.

Remedy

I ask Rachel to work at the end of the arena, away from potential distractions, and ride some walk-trot transitions. She works on a 20-meter circle, but her transitions are abrupt and disconnected, with Mucho displaying displeasure, tossing his head, and bracing against the bridle. I am convinced that by

Ride Every Step

Most of us bring less-than-ideal position habits to the saddle. I want to help you gain awareness of these bad habits and to learn ways to correct them. But, all the work you do learning the necessary skills for improved body function and balance is for naught if you don't commit yourself to focusing on the needed changes in your body while riding.

The riding environment is very challenging: You are on a moving animal! Your body's protective responses to sudden and unpredictable movement are on high alert. Unfortunately, most of these protective responses are counter to good balance and a secure position. However, through diligent practice and focus, you can make the needed changes.

A simple tool for focusing on your horse every step of the ride is to keep a metronome-like ticking in your head to match the rhythm of your horse's gait. At the walk, it is easiest to just count the hind legs' steps—otherwise the counting is too fast; at trot, count the diagonal pairs of hind leg and foreleg; at canter, count the swing of horse's hind legs as they go

Listen to Your Body

When you are already struggling with pain in your back, shoulders, hip joints, or other places, this can be aggravated by your automatic responses to the horse's sudden movement, and lead to negative tension. Many who experience pain while riding can find some comfort in an improved and stable posture (see chapter 2, p. 23). It takes a huge commitment and a great deal of focus to override your body's habits, but I know of no other more effective positive reinforcement than reducing your pain. Stay with it. You will be rewarded with more pleasurable riding, and very likely, improved performance from your horse.

Rachel anticipating that Mucho is going to become distracted, she is almost guaranteeing that it *will* happen! I urge her to focus positively on herself, her body, and the rhythm of Mucho's gaits. This helps her to think about what is actually happening *now* (not what might happen) and to ride Mucho in the way she wants him to go.

I coach Rachel through the *Rib Cage Breathing* exercises (pp. 14 and 15) while at the walk, guiding her to *inhale* (breathe in) into the lower ribs, and with each *exhale* breath to draw her core postural muscles in around her midsection. Each breath releases tension in her arms and shoulder girdle, and her contact with Mucho becomes more elastic. Her body settles into the saddle. I ask Rachel to count the steps of Mucho's *hind legs* as he lands them while walking, which will help her to focus on his movement and connect the two of them together. She carries this into walk-trot and trot-walk transitions: first counting the steps in walk, then the quicker steps in trot.

When the hay truck pulls up the driveway, Mucho stops and looks up; Rachel reacts by leaning forward and grabbing the reins with tense shoulders. She quickly recognizes her tension, so takes a breath, and gets back to riding. By taking control of her mind and body, she gains better control of Mucho and handles the distracting situation.

Exercises for Rachel: *Rib Cage Breathing 1 and 2; Bounce in Rhythm 1.*

The "Fear" Roadblock

Past riding experiences can profoundly affect your ability to commit positive focus to your ride. Memories of falls or frightening spooks can result in fear and anxiety entering your riding mindset, challenging confidence and impairing your ability to be a clear leader for your horse. Fear is a real and frustrating emotional roadblock for many riders. The psychology and treatment of fear is beyond my expertise. However, I do know that gaining confidence in your own body, through fitness and body awareness, is a positive step toward conquering anxiety. Use *Rib Cage Breathing* (see exercises on pp. 14 and 15) to find your center when your horse is tense. Count your horse's steps in every gait to stay in the moment of your ride, focusing on what is happening, rather than letting your imagination run wild, creating stories of what *might* happen.

underneath his body as the main beat of the gait (more on this in chapter 5, p. 157). Your horse will not necessarily have the ability to keep to the steadiness of a metronome, but if you focus on keeping the horse's tempo (steps per minute) as regular as possible, three things will happen: First, your focus (as it did with Rachel on p. 16) turns keenly to the present moment-by-moment movement of your horse. Second, you become much more aware that your horse's steps vary slightly but that you can also guide him to a steadier tempo. Third, by moving closely with his tempo, you become better able to influence your horse's gait in a positive way.

A Pretty Picture

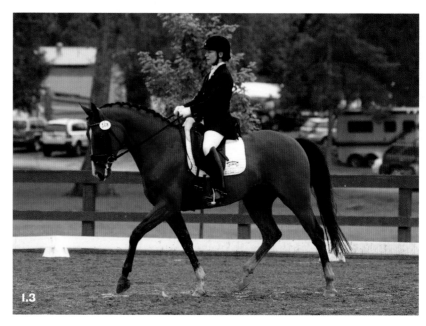

1.3

Paula Helm rides the 2005 Hungarian Warmblood gelding H.S. Whrapsody with focus and a positive "Here I am!" attitude. Paula needs to be vigilant that Whrapsody stays active and balanced in his trot. You can imagine her proactively counting his trot steps, "One-Two-One-Two" to keep them steady. As a result, she presents herself with pride and confidence—a mindset for success! Bounce in Rhythm 1 is a great exercise to perfect riding in a steady tempo.

Focusing on Your Posture Reduces Pain

Lana is a novice rider who, like many others, struggles to balance her busy work schedule with quality time with her Morgan gelding Shapiro. Her trainer rides Shapiro three times a week and Lana another three days, with one of those being a lesson. Her riding life has been further challenged by nagging back pain that her doctor ascribes to arthritis. Since her pain started, she has been limited to only riding Shapiro at the walk. Anything more causes her pain. She completed a course of physical therapy, which helped, but it has been hard for her to continue doing the prescribed exercises. Her doctor, physical therapist, trainer, and her friends all urge Lana to find a program to improve her fitness. It wasn't until she had a particularly painful ride that she realized she needed to take some time away from riding to take care of herself.

Lana starts working with me in private studio Pilates sessions. I immediately note her tendency to hold her spine in an arch. It is particularly difficult to keep her spine stable during leg exercises: The weight of her legs overwhelms her core strength and causes strain in the joints of her lower back. For several months we sort out these difficulties: She diligently does her regular exercises and, as a result, becomes much stronger and stable through her spine.

Lana returns to riding but finds it exceedingly difficult to keep herself focused on postural changes; her challenge is not a lack of strength but rather keeping her body position on her "radar" during each step of the ride. "As soon as I sit in the saddle," she says, "it is all about the horse."

Remedy

I work with Lana a few times on horseback to find ways to help her maintain her stability. As soon as she gathers up her reins, however, her spine arches forward, and her knees pull upward in the saddle, adding strain to her back. We work at the halt and review *Rib Cage Breathing* to allow her abdominal muscles to support her pelvis in the saddle. As expected, this shifts her weight in the saddle toward her tailbone. I urge her to keep that feeling and not let it change—no matter what. Repeated rib cage breaths support her spine and help her to lock in the feeling.

But back at walk—and again, as she gathers her reins—her spine alignment changes. "Where is your weight?" I ask.

"Oh!" she says, "it is too far forward!"

"That's right," I say, "Engage your abdominal muscles and change where you feel your weight in the saddle. Then stay there! This position of your pelvis and spine is so important for you. Of all the things you have to think about while you are riding, this is one detail you must not forget. You need to do this to prevent more pain."

After 30 minutes at the walk with a few walk-and-trot transitions, Lana is completely exhausted. Not physically, but mentally. Her back, however, feels fine.

Lana is an example of a fairly common phenomenon. Although you get stronger to improve your riding, that is the relatively easy part; changing your body's habits is much more difficult: It is a *mental* challenge and requires you to focus on your body position every step.

Exercises for Lana: *Rib Cage Breathing 1 and 2; Pelvic Rocking on Ball: Front to Back; Abdominal Curls*.

The following exercise, *Bounce in Rhythm,* allows you to practice keeping a steady tempo in your body. You might find it remarkably challenging to keep your body in a steady beat. But practicing this skill and gaining the awareness of

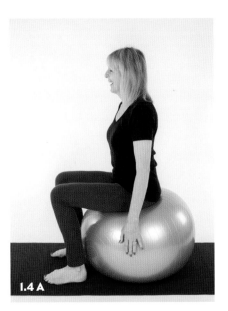

1.4 A

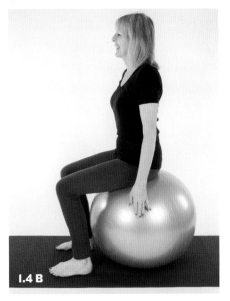

1.4 B

A Pretty Picture

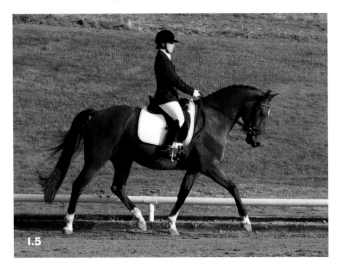

1.5

Jessica Rattner rides the 2002 Dutch Warmblood gelding Vaantje Pompen (aka "V," owned by Tamy Ryan) with focus and correct posture. Jessica describes this horse as "sensitive but opinionated." So for her to be successful, she must be clear and tactful. She does this with a stable body position that allows control of her aids. This good posture helps her feel his every move so she can respond with tact. Exercises Bounce in Rhythm 1–4 will help your ability to stay organized and in balance while moving with your horse.

how easily the tempo of your body's bouncing changes will improve both your ability to focus and the steadiness of your horse's gaits.

Bounce in Rhythm 1

To bring precision to your perception of tempo; it is a great warm-up exercise.

1 Set a metronome to 96 beats per minute.

2 Sit on an exercise ball in an upright posture and bounce on the ball in time with the metronome (figs. 1. 4 A & B).

3 Work to control your tempo so that you stay precisely with the beat. You'll find it is not as easy to do as it sounds: It is challenging to keep absolutely steady. This practice on the ball will help you guide your horse to a steady tempo.

4 Work to land the same way on the ball each time. This is also harder than it sounds, but it will help you develop skills to keep a steady position on your moving horse.

A Pretty Picture

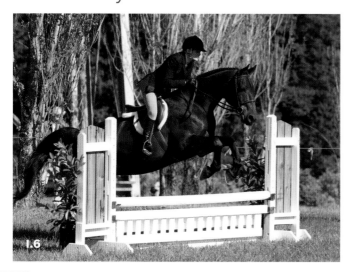

Mary Cox rides the 1979 Hanoverian mare Fatima in a hunter class in 2002. This photo was taken at Mary's first jumping show and she was terribly nervous. Knowing that her solid, schoolmaster horse would take care of her was not enough. Mary used quiet breathing to settle before entering the show ring. This helped her stay focused and ride the course fence by fence, forgetting about the crowd and the "electric" environment around her. A championship ribbon was her reward! Use Rib Cage Breathing to help your anxious mind quiet down and focus during competitions or before any ride.

Problem Solving with Focus

Keen focus on yourself and on your horse will help you solve problems that come up during your ride. Start by becoming aware of what is happening. For instance, let's say you are having trouble getting left-lead canter. Ask yourself:

"Am I truly mentally committed to going into the canter?"

"Am I afraid and being vague with my aids?"

"Am I in correct balance, or have I resorted to my bad riding habits?"

"Have I prepared my horse properly? Did I have suitable impulsion?"

Unless you focus your attention on what you are doing, it is hard to figure out the likely cause of any problem, and you risk repeating it over and over.

With your mind now engaged on movement, next I'll pursue the specifics of posture and spine alignment, which are the basics of a correct and functional riding position.

MY CHALLENGE |||||||||||||||||||||||||||||||||||||||||||||||||||||||||||||||||||||||||||||||||||||||||||||

Learning to Focus Inward

Mindful exercise has taught me how to turn my focus inward in order to feel what happens when I move. Before, when I lifted weights or did a leg exercise, it would just be about the arms lifting weights or the legs pressing a bar. With practice, though, I could feel the coordination that happened in my body to accomplish an arm or leg movement. With this awareness, movement became more balanced and fluid, and less jerky and disruptive. And, movement done with this awareness was less likely to bother my back.

This inward focus translates to my riding: With awareness I notice how my body moves on the horse, at times in undesirable ways both for my horse—and for my back. Awareness has improved my balance and timing so I can stay with my horse and give subtle aids rather than ones that are jerky and disruptive—to both of us.

2 Proper Posture

The second Rider Fundamental is *Proper Posture*: the basis for a balanced, stable, and effective riding position. Correct posture provides the foundation for efficient riding and organized management of the horse's energy. While proper posture creates an elegant position, it is not just about looking good: Good posture is a healthy position for the spine and the position from which you can most easily balance and move with efficiency.

The exercises in this chapter focus on understanding and maintaining good posture. From this stable body position, muscle suppleness in the shoulder, arm, hip joint, and leg is possible, allowing clear communication with your horse.

What Is Balance?

Balance describes a state of equilibrium, or stability and steadiness, which is maintained despite movement. Life experience teaches us how to deal with "unbalancing" situations, such as walking on rough ground, carrying an infant with one arm, or putting on a shoe while standing. When riding, however, you are expected to sit "quietly" on a constantly moving surface—the horse! Moreover, that "surface" does not always move predictably; it is no wonder that many find maintaining their balance, and coordinating their aids, extremely challenging. The moving horse presents a huge threat to balance. A sudden spook can overwhelm the balance of even the best riders and lead to a fall, but failures in balance can occur even during planned movements and transitions.

The balanced rider seeks her own "self-carriage," with her torso steadily positioned over the horse's movement; this balance must be so secure that the rider feels like a legless doll in the saddle. As mentioned, from this place, suppleness in the hip and shoulder joint muscles is possible, and the ideal image of horse and rider moving as one can emerge.

Riding in balance confers a sense of being centered, *physically* and *mentally.*

Being Physically Centered

Being *physically centered* means riding with the middle of your body as your base of support. It means riding with correct posture and postural support, and with movement controlled from the area around your center of gravity.

A concrete way to define your balanced center is to equate it to the physical location of your center of gravity. The center of gravity is a theoretical place

A Pretty Picture

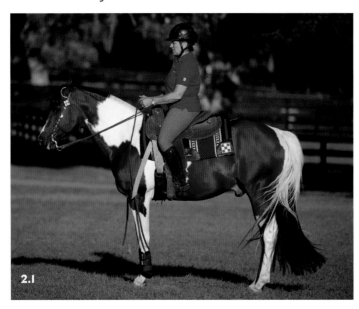

2.1

Lynn Palm, experienced English and Western trainer, shows correct neutral spine alignment (see p. 27) in Western tack aboard Rugged Painted Lark, a 1997 APHA horse she co-owns with Heidi Burkhalter. Note that Lynn's rib cage is balanced over her pelvis and she allows the normal curves of her spine. This supports a quiet, balanced halt in her horse. It doesn't matter your type of saddle, correct posture is universal to all riding disciplines! Achieve your correct posture with Find Neutral Spine and Pelvic Rocking Supine.

in the body where body weight is concentrated, or evenly distributed. In the upright human, this point is in the middle of the torso: Roughly, it's in the abdominal region just above the pelvis and a little below the belly button. For my discussion, the precise location of the center of gravity is academic; what is much more important is being able to recognize the power of riding from this general place within your body. This place should be the starting point for your aids, assisted by your arms and legs.

The stable position of your torso with muscular support around your center of gravity facilitates your center to be your *movement (kinetic) energy processing center. Energy* from your horse moving underneath you is put into your body. Learning to ride is the process of learning how to handle this energy.

First, your goal is to not fall off. Then, you strive to move with the horse and not interfere with him. Finally, you learn how to feed this energy back into the horse to direct his way of going (more forward, more up, sideways).

That the horse puts movement energy in your body is clear if you consider what happens when that energy changes: For instance, if you are not prepared, you'll fall forward during the abrupt change of movement energy inherent when going from trot to halt. And many riders find it very challenging to not have the movement energy that can come from a "large" trot send them right off their horse!

Directing your horse by considering how the center of your body interfaces with his movement energy will help you balance and do so in such a way that you will feel you are moving *with* your horse, not just sitting on top of him. You are "owning" every step of the ride. This idea, fundamental to the exercise program I present in this book (see Suggested Workouts, p. 203), inspired the Energy Management Diagram (fig. 2. 2).

For many people, accessing and riding from this processing center is not a natural or instinctive way to think of riding. Instead, it needs to be learned. This is not surprising, however, as our hand-eye-dominated life tends to draw

2.2 *This diagram shows a simple way to think of how the "movement energy" from the horse interfaces with your body. Energy comes from the horse and passes through your rider's center. You can then direct the energy forward, upward, or sideways. Using the image of this diagram will help you feel part of the horse's movement energy. Remember, however, that the stability and integrity of the torso of the rider is needed to effectively manage this energy.*

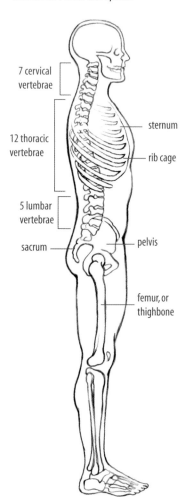

2.3 *Alignment of the vertebrae in the spine, standing. Note the curves in the seven vertebrae that comprise the neck or cervical spine; the 12 vertebrae of the thoracic spine (ribs attached); and the five vertebrae of the lumbar spine. The spine ends at the sacrum. Proper posture allows for these curves in the spine.*

7 cervical vertebrae

12 thoracic vertebrae

sternum

rib cage

5 lumbar vertebrae

sacrum

pelvis

femur, or thighbone

us away from our body's movement processing center, allowing the brain and upper body to control and dominate movement. When this happens, it leads to a stiff rider position, with shoulders and arms taking over.

But, when you keep movement control in your center, you enjoy improved balance, coordination, and grace. Consider a ballerina: Her centered movement allows extreme precision of balance so she can remain tall and steady on the toes of one foot, while creating graceful arcing movements with her arms. This is only possible with a foundation of balance from her center.

Being Mentally Centered

A correct, stable posture has the additional benefit of conferring a powerful sense of *self*, the *mental* aspect of being balanced and centered. From here, you can become a proactive rider, creating the ride you want rather than just reacting to your horse. Your center can also be a place of peace in your body. Rib cage breathing, as already discussed on page 12, draws your focus to this center. Breathing in this way helps to quiet a busy mind, allowing you to focus on your ride.

In order to find good posture and become centered and balanced on horseback, you need an understanding of basic anatomy—just enough to help you find your correct spine alignment and support it with the muscular tools within your body. So, on the following pages I will talk about the anatomy of your spine and pelvis, as well as the surrounding muscles. Throughout, I'll present exercises to improve your awareness of spine alignment and to strengthen muscles that support posture—known as the "core" muscles.

Anatomy of Posture

The Bones

Posture refers to the alignment of the spine; good posture is correct spine alignment. The spine is a series of stacked bones, known as vertebrae. It extends from the base of the skull to the sacrum, and among other functions, it provides the rigid support of our upright body position. The drawing on page 26 (fig. 2.3) shows that these vertebrae are not stacked in a straight line, but actually form curves. Seven vertebrae form a curve at the neck (cervical spine); 12 form a curve at the mid back (thoracic spine) where the ribs are attached; and five form a curve at the lower back (lumbar spine). The bottom five vertebrae of the spine are fused to form the sacrum, which is the back part of the pelvis. While the precise degree of spine curvature varies from person to person, allowing and supporting these curves preserves proper spine function and health. This alignment is called *neutral spine alignment* and it defines correct posture, which is the basis of a correct position in the saddle (see fig. 2.4 and "A Pretty Picture," p. 24).

    Neutral spine is the most efficient alignment of your spine for balance. Stated another way, if you are not in neutral spine alignment, your body must compensate somehow for your less-than-ideal posture, which can cause unnecessary and potentially harmful tension in your shoulders, back, and/or legs.

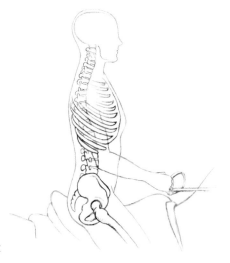

2.4 *Proper spine alignment (posture) in the saddle. Note that the curves in the neck, thoracic area, and lumbar spine are preserved, and the rider's rib cage is aligned over the pelvis.*

Vertebrae

Each vertebra of the spine has a cushioning disc between it and its neighbors above and below (fig. 2.5). These discs, as well as other bony joint connections between vertebrae, allow movement so you can rotate your spine, as well as bend it forward, backward, and sideways. However, these joints become stressed and worn out with repeated and/or excess movement, or prolonged periods of time in a posture other than neutral

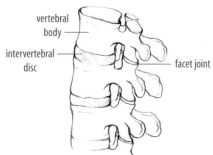

vertebral body
intervertebral disc
facet joint

2.5 *Detailed anatomy of a segment of the spine that shows the intervertebral discs and the joints between the vertebrae—common sites of inflammation and back pain.*

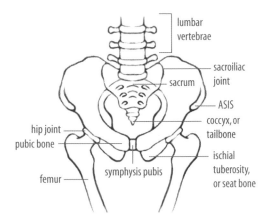

2.6 *Essentially, the pelvis is a ring of bone that connects the single column of stacked vertebrae to the legs.*

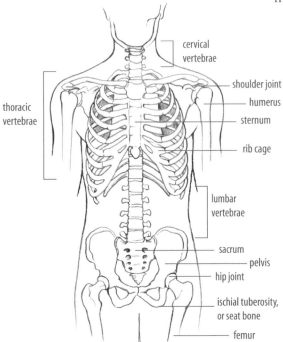

2.7 *The ribs attach to the thoracic vertebrae; the spine ends in the sacrum, which forms the back of the pelvis; the pelvis disperses the weight of the body onto the legs at the hip joints, and also disperses the concussion of walking.*

spine alignment. Back pain or nerve impingement can result. So good posture not only is beautiful and elegant, but it also helps preserve the health of your spine.

The Pelvis and Rib Cage

The spine ends in five fused vertebrae that form the sacrum—or the back of the pelvis. The *pelvis*, for our purposes, should be considered a ring of bone that connects the trunk of the body to the legs (fig. 2.6). The pelvis provides support for your abdominal and pelvic organs, and via the hip joints, disperses the downward force of your body weight onto the legs, and also absorbs concussion from the contact of your legs to the ground. The *seat bones (ischial tuberosities)* form the base—the lowest part—of the pelvis. These are the bony prominences that you sit on and are most obvious when you are on a hard chair. When in neutral spine in the saddle, the seat bones point roughly downward. The bony prominences of the right and left sides of the pelvis in the front of the body are called the *anterior superior iliac spines* (ASIS). I refer to this part of the pelvis as the ASIS in some of the exercises ahead.

In the saddle, you sit on your pelvis. The bottom of the pelvis, the pelvic floor, is what contacts the saddle. The pelvic floor consists of the muscles and tissues through which the urethra, vagina, and anus pass. The pelvic floor is shaped somewhat like a diamond, with the arch of the pubic bone in front, the sacrum (tailbone) at the back, and a seat bone on either side. The precise location of your body weight over the pelvic floor will depend upon your unique anatomy, the shape of the twist of your saddle, and your horse's anatomy. When you are in neutral spine alignment in the saddle, there is a unique distribution of weight over your pelvic floor. When there is an

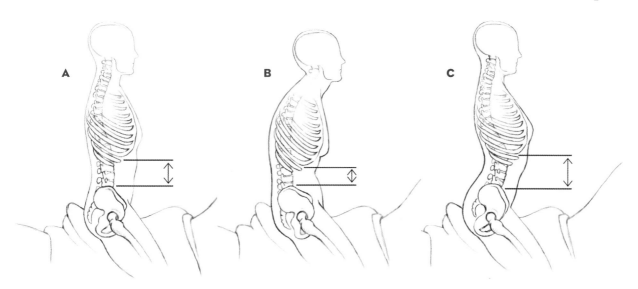

2.8 A–C *In A, neutral alignment has a defined distance between the ribs and pelvis. You can feel this distance by placing your thumb on your rib cage and your little finger on the prominent bone on the front of your pelvis, known as the ASIS. In this way, your hand is a caliper measuring this distance. When this distance remains the same while you are riding, you know your spine alignment is stable.*

In B, a rounded, or flexed, posture results in a decreased distance between ribs and pelvis in front of the body compared to neutral spine alignment. With your "hand caliper" on the front of your body, feel how this distance shortens when you bend forward in spine flexion.

In C, an arched, or extended, posture results in an increased distance between ribs and pelvis in front of the body compared to neutral spine alignment. With your "hand caliper" on the front of your body, feel how this distance lengthens when you arch your spine in extension.

alteration of this weight distribution during a ride, you know that there have been changes in your body position and alignment, hence balance.

The rib cage provides bony protection for our vital organs, the heart and lungs (fig. 2.7). The ribs connect to the thoracic vertebrae in the spine (see fig. 2.3, p. 26).

The relationship between the pelvis and rib cage in the front of the body can provide important landmarks for spine alignment. Any change in spine alignment will, by definition, alter the distance between the rib cage and the pelvis (figs. 2.8 A–C). This is most easily detected in the front of the body by considering the distance between your bottom ribs and the ASIS: When you maintain neutral spine alignment while moving or riding, this distance will stay fairly stable, but if the spine alignment changes, this distance also changes.

It takes some time and practice to understand where neutral spine alignment is in your body and what it feels like while riding. First, figure out what it feels like when you are on the ground, then, with mirrors or with feedback from someone, learn what it feels like when on your horse (see exercises beginning on p. 30). Neutral spine on horseback puts your body in the correct shoulder-hip (pelvis)-heel alignment referred to in many discussions of rider position, and it is the anatomical basis for this ideal position.

Find Neutral Spine

By lying on the floor, you can feel the alignment of the vertebrae and perceive the normal curves in your spine.

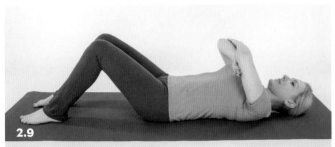

2.9

1 Lie on the floor or a mat, knees bent, feet flat on the floor, hip-joint width apart (fig. 2.9). You can rest your arms by your sides (this model has her arms folded for clarity).

2 Release the muscles of your back and let the weight of your body sink onto the floor (without pressing or forcing any part of your back onto the floor).

3 Note where you feel the weight of your body touching the floor. When the spine is in neutral alignment with its normal curves, the weight contacts the floor in three places: at the back of your pelvis (sacrum), around your shoulder and shoulder blades, and at the back of your head. There is usually little weight contacting the floor behind your waist and your neck.

This exercise describes the normal curves of your spine. Everyone is slightly different, but the point is that your back is not completely flat.

Pelvic Rocking Supine

To explore changing your spine alignment with small movements of your pelvis.

1 Lie on the floor or a mat, knees bent, feet flat on the floor, hip-joint width apart, in neutral alignment (fig. 2.10 A).

2 Take an easy *inhale* breath, breathing into your lateral rib cage.

3 On the *exhale* breath, scoop in your abdominal muscles to move the top of your pelvis toward the floor (posterior pelvic tilt or pelvic tuck) flattening your lower back (fig. 2.10 B).

4 On the next *inhale* breath, move the top of your pelvis away from the floor (anterior pelvic tilt), arching your back slightly so that your lower back comes off the floor (fig. 2.10 C).

5 Slowly alternate flattening and arching your lower back 6 to 8 times, *inhaling* as you arch your spine, *exhaling* as you flatten your spine onto the floor.

6 Gradually decrease your range of motion until, like a pendulum moving more and more slowly, your lower back comes to rest. This position is likely very close to your *neutral spine alignment.*

7 When your spine is in neutral alignment, the plane defined by three points—your pubic bone and the ASIS on the right and left sides of your pelvis—will be parallel to the floor. When you stand, or sit in the saddle, this plane is perpendicular to the floor.

Once you have found neutral spine alignment, you need to keep your spine in this position despite being on a moving horse! Support of good posture on horseback not only keeps your spine in a healthy position but also provides the most efficient position from which to achieve balance.

Next, I will look at the array of muscles around your midsection that support your posture. Often referred to as your "core" muscles, these muscles of the abdomen and back provide elastic support of spine alignment. Engaging these muscles stabilizes your posture.

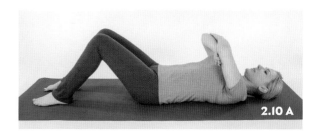

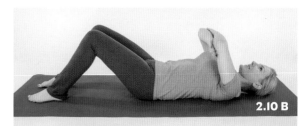

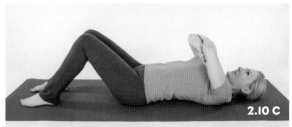

2.10 A-C *Photo A shows neutral spine alignment—the normal curves of the spine are allowed. A plane defined by the model's right and left ASIS (the front prominent part of the pelvis) and pubic bone is parallel to the floor.*

Photo B shows a posterior pelvic tilt, or pelvic tuck, with the spine rounded in flexion. The back is now flat on the floor; there is no space between the lower back and the mat. A plane defined by the model's right and left ASIS and pubic bone slopes toward the model's waist.

Photo C shows an anterior pelvic tilt with the spine arched in extension. The space between the lower back and the floor is greater than in Photo A. A plane defined by the model's right and left ASIS and the pubic bone slopes toward the model's pubic bone.

Muscles

Postural support comes from the deepest layers of abdominal and back muscles of the torso. These muscles are designed to support your upright posture throughout daily activities and to do so quite efficiently. These muscles, part of a group of muscles in our body referred to as *slow-twitch* muscles, have a metabolism that supports a low level of constant activity for prolonged periods. Their metabolic machinery works at a steady rate, using oxygen efficiently to fuel their daylong work. This makes them different from the *fast-twitch* muscles in our body, which are designed to work at high levels of activity for short periods of time.

Balance, an integral part of our daily lives (but often taken for granted), relies upon a constant low level of support from your slow-twitch, efficient postural muscles. Running for the bus, on the other hand, relies on the fast-twitch, sprinting muscles of your legs. (Consider the fatigue you experience from sprinting: Fast-twitch muscles get this job done, but at a price!) While riding, for balance we need to access the efficient postural muscles, not the fatigue-inducing leg muscles. It is the postural muscles that you access when guided to "Engage your core!" or "Stabilize your torso!" And, these are the muscles engaged during *Rib Cage Breathing* (pp. 14 and 15) to enhance the stability of your posture and balance.

The postural muscles of the torso include the deep abdominal muscles and the deep back muscles.

Abdominal Muscles

There are four layers of muscles in the abdominal wall. From deep within the body to the more superficial, they include the *transversus abdominis*, the *internal obliques*, the

Shouldn't My Back Be Flat?

I frequently encounter clients who assume that the best position of their spine is "flat," that is, without a curve in the lumbar region of the spine. This is a misunderstanding of correct posture, and emphasizes how important it is to use words precisely.

Most of us got endless cues in grade school to "Sit up straight!" Often this command stems from us rounding our shoulders forward, so the words refer to just the upper body. However, taken literally, "straight" means that we would have to counteract the normal curves of our spine.

Some of us have also been taught that when we lie flat on the floor, our lower back (lumbar spine) should contact the floor. This would again flatten out the lumbar curve and take the spine out of *neutral alignment*.

Contemporary teaching of spine alignment disagrees with flattening the back. The ideal position of your spine allows its normal curves. In this position, your body weight is distributed evenly over the body of each vertebra, allowing the cushioning disc between each vertebra to do its job of absorbing movement energy and protecting the joints in our spine.

external obliques, and the *rectus abdominis*. The first two deepest layers of abdominal muscles are the most important for *postural support*.

The *transversus abdominis* muscle fibers run transversely, that is, *across* the body (fig. 2.11). Since muscle fibers only shorten when they contract, using this abdominal muscle results in a pulled-in abdominal wall or belly, making your midsection flat. It pulls your middle to a smaller diameter—just like when you are trying to fit into jeans a size too small! Because this muscle essentially wraps all around the midsection, activating it creates a corset-like support of your spine and torso. It is the primary muscle activated in the *Rib Cage Breathing 1* and *2* exercises described in chapter 1. Pulling in the abdominal muscles on the exhale breath activates this transversus abdominis muscle and stabilizes the spine, your posture, and balance, preparing you for the next moment of your ride.

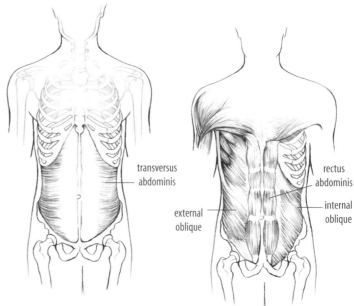

2.11 *The transversus abdominis muscle is the deepest abdominal wall muscle. Its action pulls the abdominal wall flat and is important for postural support.*

2.12 *The internal oblique, external oblique, and rectus abdominis muscles. The obliques rotate, side bend, and forward bend (flex) the trunk.*

The *internal oblique* is the second deepest muscle layer and one of three muscles shown in figure 2.12. Its fibers run from the rim of the pelvis to the rib cage. When just the right or left internal oblique muscle contracts, you will side bend or rotate to that side. When both right and left internal oblique muscles contract, they, along with the *external oblique* muscles, pull the rib cage closer to the pelvis, causing flexion (forward bending) of the spine.

The most superficial abdominal muscle, the *rectus abdominis,* is less important. This muscle, when developed, creates the "washboard abs" appearance. While some may desire this look, development of this muscle does little for posture, body support, or balance.

Back Muscles

The deep muscles of the back are as important for postural support and balance as the deep abdominal muscles. There are many layers of back muscle (fig. 2.13). The deepest layers, the *multifidi*, span only one or two vertebrae. Back-muscle activation pulls the spine into an arch, or extension.

Muscles Create a "Corset" of Support for Posture

From these muscle descriptions you can imagine how balanced use of the transversus abdominis, internal obliques, and the deep back muscles work together to move your spine in all directions, as well as to stabilize your spine in good posture despite movement forces from all directions. Like a corset around your middle, when these stabilizing muscles are engaged, they create a toned elastic support system to preserve alignment of your spine. This muscular support provides the tool for body stability and balance. Your spine stays stable despite the input of movement forces from your horse.

My exercise program teaches you to access and improve function of the deep muscles of the abdomen and back and thus develop these strong and efficient tools for balance. Some exercises directly strengthen these muscles through movement, while others challenge the ability of these muscles to maintain alignment and spine stability during leg and/or arm movements. Both approaches are valuable. You develop sufficient muscle connection, strength, and coordination to stay in good posture and balance on your moving horse, and use of an arm or leg aid does not disrupt this balance. Truly independent aids are then possible.

EXERCISES to Engage Your Deep Abdominal and Back Muscles

The following exercises are simple movements that will help you connect to and feel your deep abdominal and back muscles. These exercises are not terribly difficult—they are designed to improve your awareness of your core

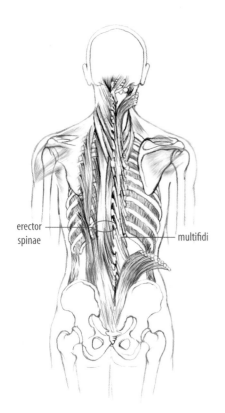

erector spinae — **multifidi**

2.13 *The back muscles cause spine extension (move the spine into an arch). The deepest layers (multifidi) are most important for spine stability.*

muscles. However, while these movements are physically straightforward, do not underestimate what they can teach you about your body. Spend time with these movements to understand how your abdominal and back muscles work together for posture. Commit unwavering focus to these movements so you can feel what is happening. The muscle skills of posture will then be more accessible to you in the saddle.

Pelvic Rocking on Ball: Front to Back
Control the position of your pelvis with your abdominal and back muscles.

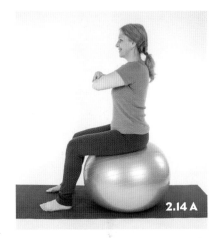

1 Sit upright (in neutral spine alignment) on an exercise ball with your feet flat on the floor hip-joint width apart (fig. 2.14 A). You may need a colleague or a mirror to check that you are in neutral spine alignment, with your shoulders aligned over your pelvis and your seat bones pointing downward.

2 Take an easy inhale breath and as you exhale, scoop in your abdominal muscles to rock your pelvis into a tuck, pointing your seat bones toward your heels and rounding your low back (fig. 2.14 B). Allow your shoulders to follow the movement; do not lean back.

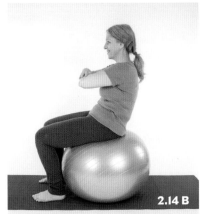

3 Inhale and use your deep back muscles to rock your pelvis back so that there is a slight arch in your spine and your seat bones point toward the back of the ball (fig. 2.14 C).

4 Exhale and tuck your pelvis under again, and inhale to point your seat bones behind you.

5 Rock back and forth between these positions 6 to 8 times, gradually settling to the middle of the movement, in neutral spine alignment.

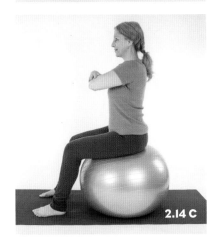

Concentrate on using your torso muscles to move your pelvis front and back. Try not to use your leg muscles to move your pelvis. This exercise should help you feel grounded, with your weight centered over your pelvis, efficiently balanced on the exercise ball.

Abdominal Curls

Strengthen your deep abdominal muscles.

1 Lie on the floor in neutral spine alignment, knees bent, feet flat on the floor hip-joint width apart.

2 Place your hands behind your head or neck.

3 Take a normal breath in and as you exhale, scoop in your lower abdomen, and peel your upper body off the floor in a curl. Inhale as you roll back down (fig. 2.15).

4 Repeat 8 to10 times.

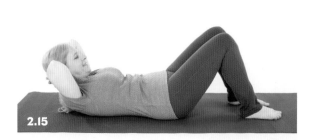

2.15

Keep your abdominal muscles scooped in as you curl up. Keep your fingers soft behind your head; don't pull yourself up with your arms. Avoid pushing your lower back into the mat by tucking your pelvis. Allow your back to lengthen. Feel your neck lengthen as you round your head forward in the curl, leading with your forehead. Curl up until just the bottom of your shoulder blades touches the floor, or less. Keep the movement smooth, not jerky. Continue breathing throughout the movement. Feel how your rib cage comes closer to your pelvis during the exercise.

Done this way, this exercise strengthens the deep abdominal muscles. If your abdominal muscles bulge out, you are using the more superficial *rectus abdominis* muscle, making the exercise less useful.

Abdominal Curls: Variation 1

Changing leg position adds difficulty to the Abdominal Curls exercise.

To make the exercise more challenging, position your legs in a tabletop position with your hip and knee joints at right angles (fig. 2.16). Perform the exercise as described above.

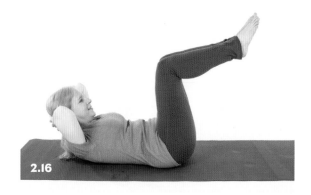

2.16

Spine Extension on Mat

This exercise strengthens the muscles of your mid and upper back.

1 Lie on the floor on your stomach, resting your forehead on a towel if needed for comfort.

2 Place your arms by your sides with palms up (fig. 2.17 A).

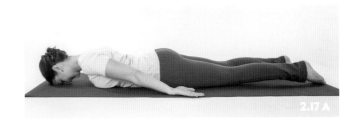

3 Take an easy inhale breath, and on the exhale breath, pull your abdominal wall up off the floor (this should not be a visible movement—just a pulling in of your abdomen to support your lumbar spine).

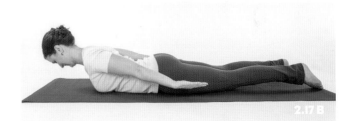

4 On the next inhale breath, bring your shoulder blades together and slowly lift your upper body off the floor. The muscles to lift your upper body should be the deep mid- and upper-back muscles (fig. 2.17 B).

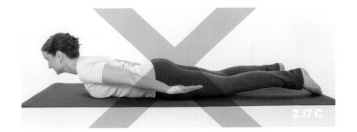

5 Exhale as you rest your upper body back down.

6 Repeat 4 to 6 times.

Initiate the movement with your shoulder blades coming down your back toward the center of your body, *not* from your neck (fig. 2.17 C). Feel that you keep your head and neck in alignment with the rest of your spine. Also feel as if your back is getting longer, reaching away from your pelvis. If this exercise causes low back pain, reduce the range of motion and seek support from your scooped-in, deep abdominal muscles, or avoid the exercise until you can get expert feedback.

Follow the exercise set with a *Back Stretch* (next).

Back Stretch

Provide relief for back muscles after they have worked.

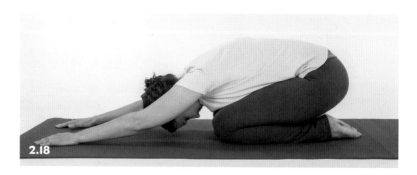

1 Start on your hands and knees. Sit back toward your heels and lower your forehead toward the mat (fig. 2.18).

2 Either reach your arms "overhead," resting your hands on the floor, or keep them by your sides.

3 Use your breath to stretch your back muscles. As you breathe in, feel how expanding your rib cage stretches your back muscles. As you exhale, focus on scooping in the abdominal muscles to support the stretch of your lower back muscles. Hold for several breaths.

4 Walk your hands over to your right side, stretching the left side of your body. Breathe into the left rib cage two to three times to facilitate the stretch.

5 Walk your hands over to your left side, stretching the right side of your rib cage. Breathe into the right rib cage.

Spine Stretch Forward

Provide a stretch to your back and improve awareness of the location of your rib cage in relation to your pelvis.

1 Sit on an exercise ball in neutral spine alignment, feet flat on the floor hip-joint width apart. Raise your arms out in front of you, parallel to the floor (fig. 2.19 A). Avoid shrugging your shoulders.

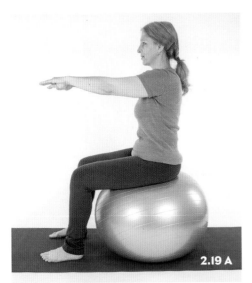 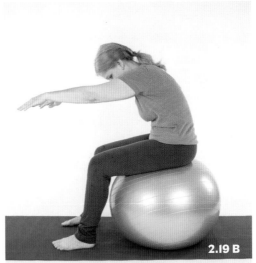

2.19 A   2.19 B

2 On an exhale breath, round your body forward over your lap, reaching forward with your arms but keeping them parallel to the floor (fig. 2.19 B).

3 Inhale while you are curled over, and on the next exhale breath, starting from the base of your spine, press your spine back onto the vertical, feeling the vertebrae in your back stack on top of each other as you return to sitting upright.

4 Repeat 3 to 5 times.

Keep your weight centered over your pelvis. In this exercise, you are not just leaning forward, you are rounding your low back over your lap. Your weight should shift only slightly onto your feet. Feel your abdominal muscles press back against your spine, giving it a stretch. Feel lifted over your lap. Imagine there is a wall behind your body—your back peels away from this wall as you round forward, and feel it return to the wall as you roll back up.

Spine Extension: Scarecrow

Activate the muscles of your upper back. (I call it the "anti-computer-posture" exercise.)

1 Sit on an exercise ball in neutral spine alignment, feet flat on the floor hip-joint width apart.

2 Lift your arms out to the side with bent elbows. Rotate your arms so that your hands reach to the ceiling: the "scarecrow" position (fig. 2.20 A).

3 Keeping your shoulder blades wide, lift your sternum up toward the ceiling by engaging the muscles of your back between your shoulder blades (fig. 2.20 B). This is a small movement; think of a slight rotation of your rib cage so that your sternum barely lifts upward. Avoid taking all of the motion in your neck and lower back (fig. 2.20 C). Keep your seat bones directly under you.

4 Hold this small thoracic extension for a few counts, and then release.

5 Repeat 3 to 5 times.

RIDER'S CHALLENGE ||||||||||||||||||||||||||||||||||||||||||||||||||||||||||||||||||||||||||||||||||||||||||||||||||||||||||||||||

Organize Riding from the Center

Stephanie, a new rider at my clinic, rides over on her spicy, 16-years-young Thoroughbred gelding, Atticus. I ask her about her lesson goals.

"I don't know," Stephanie replies. "I'm sure I need to work on a lot of things."

Stephanie moves onto the rail with high-headed Atticus and picks up a posting trot. Atticus is irregular in his tempo, causing Stephanie to alternately fall back as he moves off into his quick trot, and fall forward when he slows down in response to her pulling on the reins. This pattern gets repeated with Stephanie alternately kicking to keep him in trot, falling backward as he trots forward, then pulling on the reins to slow him down and falling forward as he does. He remains tense and snorting at the environment, while Stephanie struggles for consistency.

Remedy

Stephanie needs to gain mastery over her own focus and balance to control Atticus's trot. She must buy into riding *every step* and riding for the trot *she wants*—that is, become a *proactive*, rather than a *reactive*, rider. She must develop a clear sense of balance around her center and ride from it rather than just from her arms and legs.

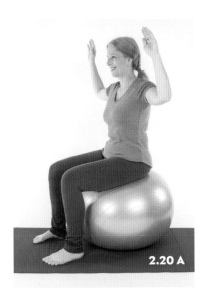 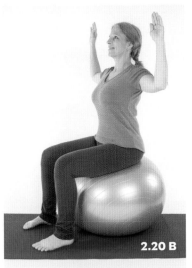 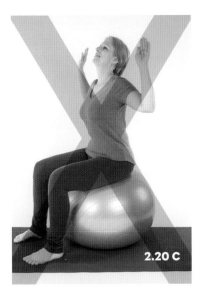

2.20 A   2.20 B   2.20 C

Note: I am not particular about the breathing with this exercise, so long as you breathe!

I find it convenient and useful to combine these last two exercises. Perform one *Spine Stretch Forward* and then one *Spine Extension: Scarecrow*. The alternate spine flexion and spine extension enhance awareness of spine alignment. (This is the sequence listed in the Suggested Workouts at the end of the book, p. 205.)

I teach Stephanie the *Rib Cage Breathing* technique so she can get a sense of her source of balance coming from the middle of her body. With one hand, I gently press against her lower abdomen, bringing her abdominal wall closer to her spine, without rounding her back. My other hand presses against her lower back to keep it in a stable position. I urge her to keep her abdominal muscles engaged and pulling inward to help stabilize her balance and to imagine there is a "hum" of energy coming from these core muscles supporting her body during the ride.

Back on the rail, Stephanie practices her breathing to engage her core muscles. She rides some walk-halt

transitions, focusing on using her breath to stabilize her body during the halt and to prepare her body to move forward with Atticus into the walk. In trot, I encourage her to keep her core muscles "humming" and to feel her center moving forward and back in the posting trot. She counts a steady tempo to stabilize her horse's tempo (see *Bounce in Rhythm 1*, p. 21). Atticus continues his speeding-up and slowing-down cycles, but Stephanie's body position stays fairly steady and her aids become less dramatic and destabilizing.

Exercises for Stephanie: *Rib Cage Breathing 1* and *2*; *Bounce in Rhythm 1*; *Pelvic Rocking on Ball: Front to Back*; *Spine Stretch Forward*; *Spine Extension: Scarecrow*.

A Pretty Picture

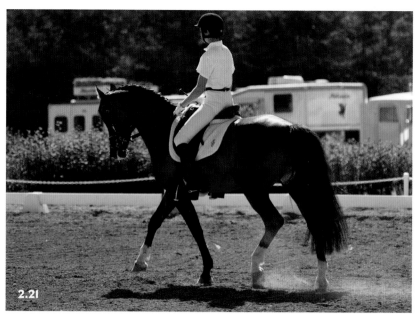

2.21

Garyn Heidemann shows organization and focus while riding the 2005 Oldenburg stallion Avatar (owned by Sheila Buchanan) down the centerline. Garyn's long torso requires her to pay special attention to her spine alignment so it does not waver from its correct position and cause this easily distracted stallion to become tense. Correctly performed Plank on Mat: Knees or Plank on Mat: Feet exercises help Garyn maintain this position.

EXERCISES to Strengthen Your Core

Now that you have a better sense of your deep abdominal and back muscles, try these more challenging exercises to further strengthen your core. Continue to apply committed focus to the exercise, and consider what is moving and working. Be vigilant about coordinating breathing with the exercises so your stabilizing *exhale* breaths work not only during exercises, but also during your ride, and during your day.

Abdominal Curls Sustained

Add more challenge to the Abdominal Curls exercises (p. 36), by performing a single sustained curl.

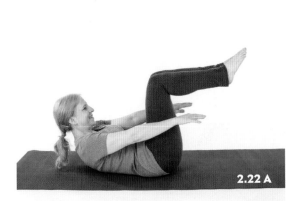
2.22 A

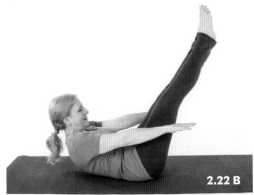
2.22 B

1 Lie on the floor in neutral spine alignment, knees bent, feet flat on the floor hip-joint width apart.

2 Place your arms by your sides.

3 Take a normal breath in and as you exhale, scoop in your lower abdomen and peel your upper body off the floor in a curl, reaching your arms forward toward your shins. Place your legs in a tabletop position *or* straighten your legs onto a high diagonal line (figs. 2.22 A & B).

4 Keep the curled position as you breathe in and out. Try to breathe into your posterior rib cage so your inhale breath does not cause you to lose any of the curl. Each time you exhale, pull your abdominal muscles inward.

5 Repeat for 8 to 10 breaths.

If your neck gets sore during the sustained curl, try to curl up a bit more, or support your head with your hands. Keep an inward pull on your abdominal muscles, and avoid letting them bulge outward. Extend your legs straight onto a high diagonal line only when your abdominal muscles are strong enough to support your lower back.

Crisscross

Another Abdominal Curls variation that puts greater demand on the oblique abdominal muscles.

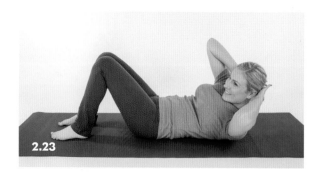

2.23

1 Lie on the floor in neutral spine alignment, knees bent, feet flat on the floor hip-joint width apart.

2 Place your hands behind your head or neck.

3 Take a normal breath in and as you exhale, scoop in your lower abdomen and peel your upper body off the floor in a curl. At the top of the curl, add a rotation of your torso to the left, as if you were bringing your right rib cage toward your left pelvis (fig. 2.23). Inhale as you roll back down.

4 Repeat the curl rotating toward the right, bringing your left rib cage toward your right pelvis.

5 Repeat 6 to 8 times each direction.

Coordinate your breath with the movement. Avoid lifting your head with your arms, but feel your abdominal muscles pull your rib cage toward your pelvis, then add the rotation from your abdominals, not your arms. The focus is on curling up and then rotating.

Crisscross Sustained

To add more challenge to the Crisscross exercise, sustain the curl.

1 Lie on the floor in neutral spine alignment, knees bent, feet flat on the floor hip-joint width apart.

2 Place your hands behind your head or neck.

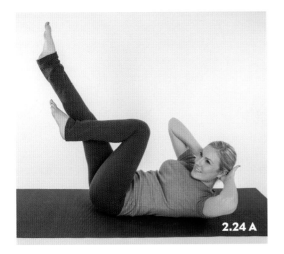

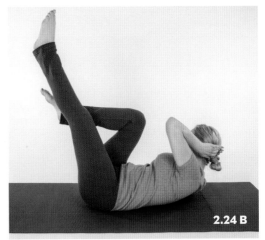

3 Take a normal breath in and as you exhale, scoop in your lower abdomen and peel your upper body off the floor in a curl. Position your right leg straight at a 45-degree angle, or high diagonal, and place your left leg in a tabletop position. Rotate your torso toward your left knee (fig. 2.24 A).

4 Reverse the leg positions and the rotation in your torso (fig. 2.24 B).

5 Breathe out each time you rotate, and breathe in as you switch your leg position.

6 Repeat 8 times in each direction.

As with the other *Abdominal Curls* exercises, avoid lifting your head and rotating your body with your arms; use your abdominal muscles to draw the rib cage to the pelvis, then to one side. Focus more on the *up* part of the curl, not the turning part of the curl. Carefully place your legs in their correct positions, feeling your straight leg reach out of the hip joint. Keep your leg position under control.

Abdominal Muscles: Pull In or Push Out?

I frequently encounter two questions about abdominal muscle function. The first is, "I'm told to push my abdomen or belly out in front of me. What does that mean?" And the second is, "I've been told to use my abdominals by pushing them out. How do I do that?"

The first question is simply one of semantics. A person with a posture that is *flexed* (also called *rounded* or a *C-shaped posture*) may be coached to correct this posture by pushing her abdomen or belly out in front to accomplish a more upright position closer to neutral spine alignment. But to me, it makes sense to address the postural issue directly and guide such a rider to use the muscles of her back to stabilize a more upright posture. I do not think the cue "Let your belly hang out in front of you" is useful, as I believe supportive tone is needed from your abdominal muscles for optimal posture and balance on a moving horse.

I teach using the deep abdominal muscles in an inward, corset-like fashion to support spine stability. Many physical therapists (see Carolyn Richardson Phd. et al.) endorse this means of dynamic spine stability. It has been demonstrated that during normal spine function, the *transversus abdominis* (a deep abdominal muscle that creates the corset around your middle), and the *multifidi* (deep spine extensor muscles) are triggered to support the spine in anticipation of movement or a load. This suggests the body's innate choice for spine stability is these muscles, which work in an inward fashion. Consciously engaging these muscles facilitates dynamic spine stability and supported movement.

Other spine experts suggest that spine stability is best accomplished by bracing the abdominal muscles outward—the same way you would during a cough, or a bowel movement. This technique of spine stability is usually recommended in the context of a brief need for spine "stiffness," such as during competitive weight lifting or delivering a karate blow to a hard surface. By pushing the abdominal muscles outward, you encase the spine in a rigid block and support the spine during the forceful movement.

Bracing the abdominal muscles outward, however, is not practical while riding for two reasons. First, this position is hard to maintain for long, and second, rigidity of the spine is not ideal in riding: There is some movement in the spine and pelvis; it makes most sense to me to find a way to keep the motion within a small range by supporting the spine with engaged muscles of the core—that is, the inward elastic tone of the deep abdominal and back muscles.

I personally have explored both methods of stabilizing torso position in the saddle. I find the inward corset approach logical, doable, and effective. What's more, this technique of core stability and support is what you see in any sport or activity that requires balance and movement. After all, you don't see ballerinas pushing out their bellies, right?

All of the core exercises thus far presented involve moving the spine. Core muscles are strengthened as the muscles shorten—abdominal muscles pulling the front of the rib cage toward the pelvis in spine flexion in the *Abdominal Curls* sequences; back muscles pulling the front of the rib cage away from the pelvis in the *Spine Extension* exercises. Finally, the diagonally placed, oblique abdominal muscles add rotation in the Crisscross exercises on pp. 44 and 45. In the saddle, however, you want stability of the spine—that is, despite changes in forward or sideways energy, you want to keep your body in a balanced upright position. Muscles that we have thus far used to move your spine will now be put to work keeping your spine alignment stable.

A Pretty Picture

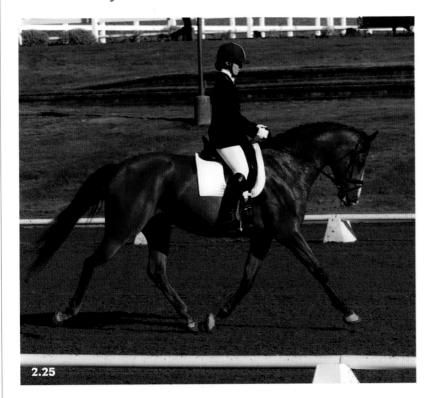

2.25

Catherine Reid riding the 2004 Swedish gelding Karibbean (owned by Carolynn Bunch) in a lengthened trot and showing good upright spine alignment. Coordinated function of her abdominal and back muscles create an elastic corset around her torso supporting this correct alignment, and it keeps Catherine aligned over Karibbean's long trot stride. This support best comes from an inward pull of the abdominal and waist muscles around Catherine's spine. Catherine notes that Karibbean's lengthened trot is quite energetic and he can tend to race. She must stay stable in her position to prevent him from quickening and running on his forehand. Useful exercises to keep with a big trot: Plank on Mat: Knees and/or Plank on Mat: Feet.

Plank on Mat: Knees

A fantastic integrating exercise for core muscles function and shoulder and leg support. Plus, it does not require equipment.

1 Lie on your stomach on a mat.

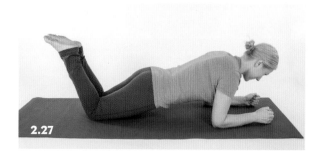

2.27

2 Bend your elbows and keep them by your sides and place your forearms on the mat. Bend your knees so your lower legs are off the floor.

3 While keeping your shoulders stable, lift yourself onto your knees and forearms into a suspended plank position (fig. 2.27). Seek a long and neutral

A Pretty Picture

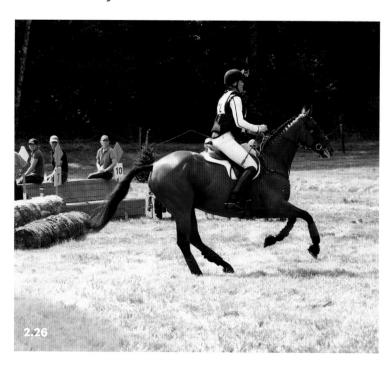

2.26

Karen O'Neal approaches a cross-country fence aboard her 2002 "off-the-track" Thoroughbred gelding Markus. Appreciate the integration of her core muscles that supports her posture, torso position, arms, and legs while she steadies Markus and helps him collect his long gallop stride in preparation for the jump. Karen's organization helps Markus develop security and confidence over fences. Should she get unbalanced (by falling to the right or left, or ahead of or behind her horse) before the fence, Markus is faced with both the challenge of the upcoming jump as well as the changing location of his rider. Karen can only keep control of her tall torso by using all her core muscles in a coordinated fashion. All integrating core exercises enhance this skill: Plank on Mat: Knees; Plank on Mat: Feet; Plank on Ball; Quadruped: Single; Quadruped: Diagonal.

spine position and avoid pulling your shoulders up around your ears. Try to keep your pelvis level, not pushed up to the ceiling.

4 Hold this position for 30 to 60 seconds.

Plank on Mat: Feet
It's a much more challenging version of *Plank on Mat: Knees.*

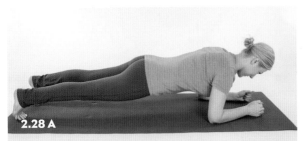

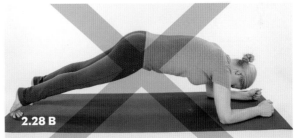

1 Lie on your stomach on a mat.

2 Bend your elbows and keep them by your sides and place your forearms on the mat. Keep your legs straight.

3 While keeping your shoulders stable, lift yourself onto your feet and forearms into a suspended plank position (fig. 2.28 A). Seek a long and neutral spine position and avoid pulling your shoulders up around your ears. Try to keep your pelvis level, *not* pushed up toward the ceiling (fig. 2.28 B).

4 Hold this position for 30 to 60 seconds.

If *Plank on Mat: Feet* is too challenging, alternate between your feet and knees for the 30 to 60 seconds of the exercise. Gradually build up the time you can hold the position on your feet. Done correctly, either plank exercise is a good integrator of abdominal and back muscles, as well as the shoulder girdle and leg muscles. When I see a rider being pulled or tossed around by her horse, I say, "Think plank!" to encourage body stability and balance.

Plank on Ball

Integrate core muscle function, with the challenge of balance offered by the ball.

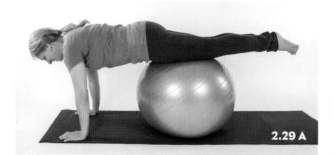
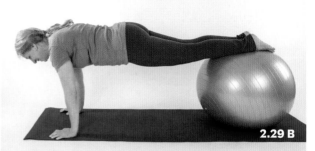

1 Lie on your stomach over an exercise ball.

2 Shift your weight toward your hands and walk your hands out onto the floor. Lift your legs up behind you so that your body is in a plank-like position, your spine in neutral alignment.

3 Begin by walking out until the front of your thighs rests on the ball (fig. 2.29 A). Hold this position for several breaths, then release back to lying on your stomach or the ball.

4 Repeat 3 to 5 times.

Keep your abdominal muscles engaged to support your back. Keep the front of your shoulders open and your shoulder blades coming back and down, without letting your back arch.

The exercise can be made more difficult by walking farther out so that the front of your knees or lower legs rest on the ball (fig. 2.29 B). The farther you move away from the ball, the more you will need support from your trunk muscles to maintain neutral alignment and secure balance.

Quadruped: Single

Maintain a stable spine position while moving an arm or a leg.

1 Start on your mat in a hands-and-knees position with knees lined up under your hip joints and hands lined up under your shoulder joints (fig. 2.30 A). (If this bothers your wrists, put your hands in a fist position.) Imagine your torso as a rectangular box; keep the shape of the box stable during the entire exercise.

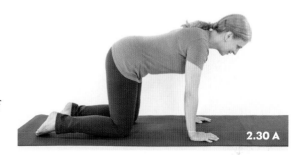

2.30 A

2 On an exhale breath, extend your right arm out in front of you just far enough to take it out of supporting your weight (fig. 2.30 B). As you inhale, bring your arm back.

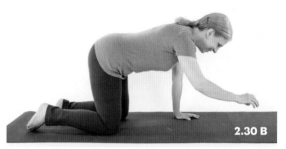

2.30 B

3 Then, again on an exhale breath, extend your left arm out and bring it back.

4 On another exhale breath, slide your right leg out behind you. You needn't lift your leg much off the ground; just remove it from is support position. "Inhale" it back into position.

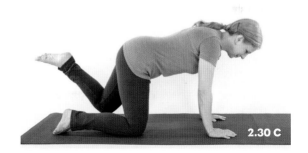

2.30 C

5 Finally, slide your left leg out behind you and inhale as you bring it back (fig 2.30 C).

6 Lift each arm and leg two to three times.

The goal during this exercise is to keep your torso as a stable rectangular box. Note how difficult it is to keep your center stable when bringing either of your legs out of support position. Try to not have your weight shift to the left as you slide your right leg back, and vice versa. This requires integration of your core stabilizing muscles. Focus on using your exhale breath as a reminder to engage the muscles of your core to keep your torso stable. Rather than your body shifting to preserve balance, your core muscles hold you still.

Quadruped: Diagonal

This more difficult version of Quadruped further challenges spine stability while you move your arms and legs.

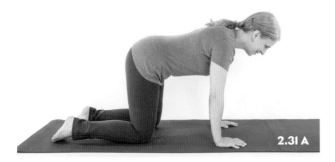

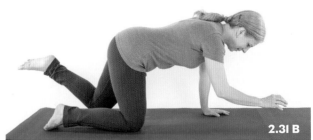

2.31 A

2.31 B

1 Start on your mat in a hands-and-knees position with knees lined up under your hip joints and hands lined up under your shoulder joints (fig. 2.31 A. (If this bothers your wrists, put your hands in a fist position.) Imagine your torso as a rectangular box; keep the shape of the box stable during the entire exercise.

2 On an exhale breath, extend your right arm out in front of you and your left leg out behind you at the same time (fig. 2.31 B). As you inhale, bring them back.

3 Repeat, extending your left arm with your right leg.

4 Lift each diagonal pair 4 to 6 times.

Avoid a large lateral shift of your weight as you lift your hand and knee off the mat. Try to keep the center of your body stable while moving your arm and leg. This takes practice. To anchor your position, focus on your core muscles.

Common Posture Challenges

Many rider-position issues have at their root a problem with posture and postural support. I have worked with hundreds of riders, and have found postural issues in over 90 percent. Some issues are small, but some contribute significantly to training difficulties.

In this book, I define ideal position in the saddle as *neutral spine alignment on the vertical.* (There are circumstances, such as the forward position for jumping, where being in front of the vertical is clearly desired, but these riders should still be in neutral spine alignment, see fig. 2.32.)

When first assessing any rider, I ask myself, "Is this rider in neutral spine alignment? If so, is she on the vertical, with shoulders balanced over the pelvis?" Until these criteria are met, it is very difficult to make lasting changes in any other rider position issue, such as an errant arm or foot. Without

Improve Your Form, Improve Your Comfort

For some riders, a faulty riding position causes them pain. When faced with a rider who finds riding to be uncomfortable, I first assess posture. Even arm or leg dysfunction and pain might have poor posture as a significant contributory factor.

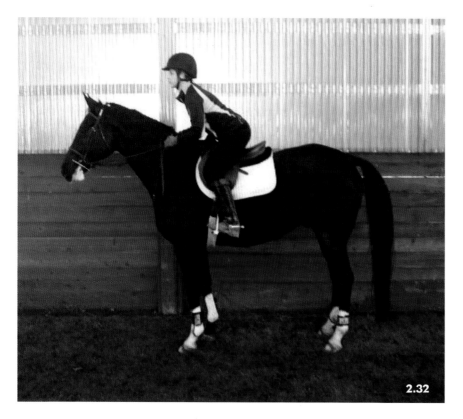

2.32

Kate Shook demonstrates a correct, neutral spine, two-point position on Lola Michelin's 2001 Hanoverian gelding Amarosso. You should keep correct alignment of the spine regardless of whether your torso position is upright or forward in two-point. The change in angle of the torso to a forward two-point position should happen from movement only at the hip joint, not by changing the alignment of the vertebrae in the spine. This requires awareness of correct neutral spine alignment, stability of posture with core muscles, and movability or suppleness at the hip joint. Useful exercises to develop these skills include Find Neutral Spine; Pelvic Rocking Supine; Pelvic Rocking on Ball: Front to Back; Plank on Mat: Knees; Plank on Mat: Feet; Knee Circles; and Leg Circles.

the basis of stable balance from proper alignment and torso support, any adjustment of arm or leg position is likely to be fleeting.

It is not unusual to see riders in fairly good spine alignment who tend to ride *behind the vertical* (leaning back). A slight leaning back position can sometimes offer extra stability for sitting trot (see chapter 5, p. 157), but it is not the best position because it can encourage the horse to come on his forehand. To repeat: Correct spine alignment on the vertical is the best position for optimum balance in the rider—and the horse.

The position and fit of your saddle can dramatically affect your ability to find correct pelvic position and, hence, spine alignment. Get help with saddle fitting if you are fighting your saddle for correct position or are concerned about how the saddle positions your body.

The Flexed (Rounded or C-Shaped) Posture

Some riders tend to adopt a *flexed* alignment of the spine while in the saddle (fig. 2.33). This puts the spine in a rounded position, or in spine flexion (forward bending). This postural problem is not uncommon in riders who spend a great deal of their day sitting in front of a computer or desk, and it creates problems both on and off the horse. It risks excess strain on the lower back because the body weight is pressing on the intervertebral discs in an uneven fashion. Riders with this posture often look down at their horse's neck. If they look up, as shown in the illustration to the left, their posture causes a shortened cervical spine with too much curve, and a jutting chin. This strains the discs and joints in the neck.

Remedy

To correct this flexed posture, increase the activity and use of your back muscles to pull your upper back to a more upright position and restore the lumbar curve of your spine (figs. 2.34 A & B). This will lengthen the too short distance between your rib cage and pelvis in the front of your body (see fig. 2.8 B, p. 29). Stretching the muscles of your shoulder girdle will also help. If this is your posture at work, take periodic stretch breaks to disrupt this harmful

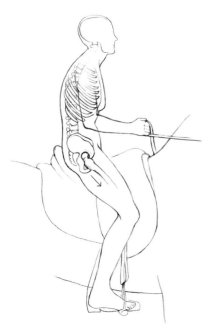

2.33 *A flexed (rounded or C-shaped) posture. The seat bones point toward the horse's shoulders (see arrow) rather than straight down; the rider's shoulders are hunched forward; and there is little or no lumbar curve in the spine.*

Correcting Flexed Posture

In A, Patty Ruemmler demonstrates a flexed (rounded) posture on her 2007 Gypsy Vanner mare Melantha (aka "Millie"). Note that her seat bones point toward Millie's shoulders, her lower back is rounded, and the front of her body is too short. Patty's feet are out in front of her and she is looking down—common characteristics of a flexed posture.

In B, Patty corrects this flexed posture by engaging the muscles of her back to pull her upper body back on the vertical. Now her seat bones point downward and she has improved balance in her core muscles. Exercises useful to correct a flexed posture include *Spine Extension: Scarecrow; Spine Extension on Mat;* and *Chest Expansion.*

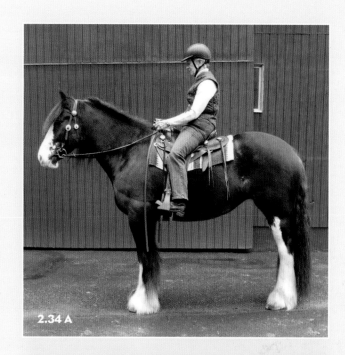

2.34 A

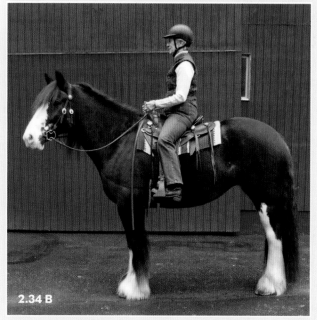

2.34 B

Consequences of Flexed Posture
Strains rider's intervertebral discs
Can lead to a chair seat with rider behind the horse's movement
Often comes packaged with rounded shoulders
Often comes packaged with a tendency to look down
"Closes off" the front of the rider's body, discouraging ground covering strides
Invites (or is caused by) overuse of the gluteal muscles
Risks rider using the reins for balance

A Pretty Picture

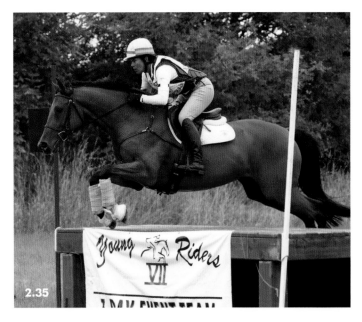

2.35

Meika Descher rides her homebred 2006 Thoroughbred/Zangersheide cross gelding DeNovo (owned by Polestar Farm) with focus and correct balance. Meika took her time bringing along this talented gelding, waiting for him to mature before entering him in many competitions. Surely her stable position has contributed to "Dino" gaining trust in her guidance. The large jump and thrust inherent in a cross-country fence can easily send a rider into a flexed (rounded) posture, but Meika maintains correct tone in her back to avoid this pitfall. Exercises that develop this skill include Spine Extension: Scarecrow and Spine Extension on Mat.

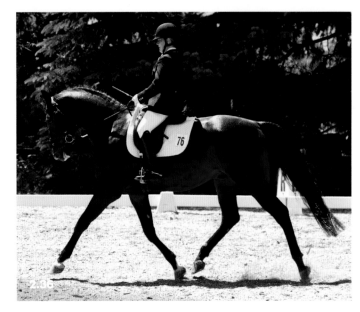

2.36

Caryn Bujnowski riding the 2001 Hanoverian gelding Dylan stays correctly upright at sitting trot, avoiding a rounded back. Caryn notes that her many years of riding young horses causes her to tend to flex (round forward) her spine so she is diligent about keeping the front of her chest open and eyes up. This strategy is needed with this powerful gelding, who, as Caryn says, "can get distracted and revert to his stallion personality if I'm not focused." Useful exercises for Caryn are: Spine Extension: Scarecrow and Spine Extension on Mat.

position. Try the *Spine Extension: Scarecrow* exercise at the computer during your workday: It does not require you to get out of your chair, but it stretches and engages muscles to counteract the tendency to round forward while typing and looking at the computer screen—and it requires *no* equipment.

Take time to break this postural habit when you ride, too. This takes great focus because it is very challenging to expect your body to adopt a posture in

RIDER'S CHALLENGE ||||||||||||||||||||||||||||||||||||||||||||||||||||||||||||||||||||||||||||||||||||||||||||||||

A Flexed (Rounded or C-Shaped) Posture

Julie asks for help with balance on her big-moving Hanoverian gelding, Bismark. Despite a full-time work schedule, she manages to ride about four days a week—and she does so with great focus and commitment.

Bismark moves off in his lanky trot. His attitude is one of "I do just enough to get by." The two of them appear "earthbound," needing to work hard against gravity. In the down phase of the posting trot, Julie lands heavily behind Bismark's movement with a flexed posture, her legs too far in front of her. She struggles to keep Bismark in the trot and tries to push him forward each time she lands in the saddle by squeezing her gluteal muscles. She sets up a cycle of kicking him forward but falling behind him in a flexed posture. Bismark carries on in a blasé manner.

Two issues contribute to Julie's difficulty keeping Bismark in an active trot: her posture, and her leg position and function. (Read more about how we resolve Julie's leg position and function problems in chapter 3, p. 116.)

Julie's flexed posture puts her center of gravity behind Bismark's and blocks him from moving forward. When she is behind his motion, her body is telling him to slow down, which she most certainly does not want. Her flexed posture makes it nearly impossible for her to come to a proper balance point in the posting trot; she is always a bit behind him.

Remedy

At the halt, I have Julie do some forward and backward *Pelvic Rocking* exercises in the saddle to show how she places too much weight in the posterior (toward the tailbone) part of her pelvic floor. I move Julie's spine closer to neutral alignment by having her slightly arch her back, restoring her lumbar curve. This engages her back muscles, adjusts her pelvis so that her seat bones point downward, and releases her gluteal muscles. I have Julie make a mental note of where she feels her weight distribution over her pelvic floor. I also adjust her leg position so that her feet come back underneath her, creating the correct shoulder-hip (pelvis)-heel line.

Julie picks up the posting trot. Bismark is reluctant. Julie kicks harder, slipping into her flexed posture and falling behind his movement. Bismark, of course, slows down. I coach her to a better posture, which keeps her in balance and confers a "Let's go!" attitude to her horse. Bismark responds by offering a longer stride. Julie struggles to break the habit of giving a leg aid every step, rounding her back, squeezing her gluteal muscles, and falling behind the movement. But when she keeps her spine aligned correctly and her feet underneath her, her balance improves; the two of them no longer appear earthbound, but rather in self-carriage, moving forward.

Exercises: *Pelvic Rocking on Ball: Front to Back; Spine Extension on Mat; Spine Extension: Scarecrow; Pelvic Bridge: Simple.*

the saddle that is different from your "norm." This flexed (rounded, C-shaped) posture often comes packaged with the habit of overusing the gluteal (butt) muscles to aid the horse. These muscles can pull the pelvis into a tuck, contributing to flattening the low back. I have found that using the gluteal muscles while riding should be reserved for a few rare circumstances; many riders overuse these muscles and suffer compromised posture and hip-joint mobility as a result (see chapter 3, p. 90).

A flexed posture can also be seen in a fearful rider who adopts a fetal position when the horse moves unpredictably. Unfortunately, this response is counterproductive and creates a less stable base of support and balance. Exact management of such a situation must be considered individually and is beyond the scope of this discussion. However, learning good posture and postural support in and of itself can do wonders to improve your confidence in your own body and, hence, confidence in the saddle.

Extended (Arched) Posture

While some riders struggle to correct a *flexed (rounded or C-shaped)* posture, even more ride with an *extended (arched)* posture. Sometimes, in an effort to "sit up straight with shoulders back," a rider develops too much tone in the mid- and upper-back muscles. This pulls the spine into an arch (fig. 2.37). As you will see in "The Rider's Challenge" on p. 60, this tension can spread to the arms and limit suppleness of the shoulder muscles, compromising contact with the horse through the bridle. This postural problem is an important cause of a "tense" or "stiff" appearance. Further, an extended posture puts excess strain on the facet joints between each vertebra of the spine.

Remedy

Using the abdominal muscles to both pull the rib cage slightly closer to the pelvis in the front of the body and lift the pubic bone up toward the sternum will correct this posture (figs. 2.38 A & B). It takes some focus to make this change; I encourage riders to feel a constant "hum" of their abdominal muscles

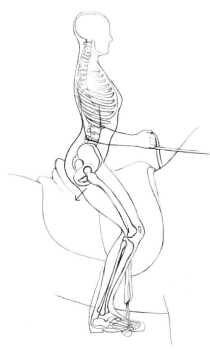

2.37 *An extended (arched) posture. The seat bones point toward the horse's back legs rather than straight down (see arrow); there is too much curve in the lumbar spine; and the shoulders are tight.*

Correcting Extended Posture

In A, Kirsten Miller demonstrates an incorrect extended (arched) posture on her 1998 Norwegian Fjord mare Bergen Saundra. Notice that the front of her torso is too long, and her back is short and contracted. Her seat bones point backward toward Bergen's hind legs. Kirsten finds herself stuck in this extended posture on Bergen sometimes, especially if the mare gets a little strong in the bridle. However, Kirsten recognizes that arching her back can encourage Bergen to travel on her forehand, and risks straining Kirsten's back.

In B, Kirsten corrects this posture by bringing her ribs and pelvis closer together in the front of her body. *Pelvic Rocking: Front to Back* and *Abdominal Curls* help her to develop the awareness and muscle tone to prevent an extended posture.

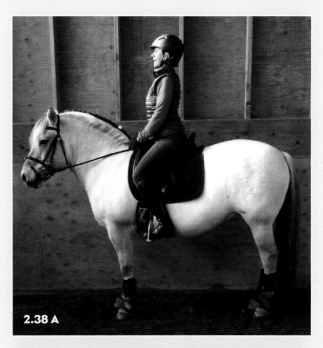

2.38 A

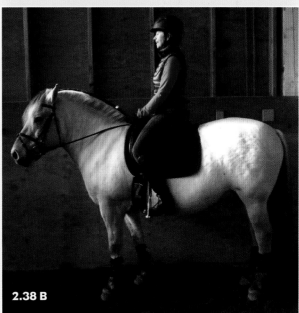

2.38 B

Consequences of Extended Posture
Causes rider to appear tense and feel unstable
Limits suppleness in the shoulder girdle
Makes it hard to find elastic contact
Pulls rider's focus up and away from center of gravity
Encourages riding from shoulders and hands, not from the center of the body
Creates precarious balance
Causes low- or mid-back pain
Places strain on facet joints of the spine
Perches rider *on top of* the horse, not sitting and moving *with* the horse

Extended (Arched) Posture

Melissa nervously enters the arena, matching the mindset of her mare, Belle, a 12-year-old Arab/Thoroughbred cross. I ask how I might help her.

"I carry tension in my shoulders," she answers as Belle scurries off in a rapid walk.

I watch Melissa and Belle warm up at walk, trot, and canter. Melissa carries her body in a tense, upright fashion, with her shoulders living up around her ears. Her spine is extended (arched) so that her seat bones point back toward the horse's hind feet, and her upper body tends to pitch forward. Belle trots around with quick, short steps, avoiding contact with the bit.

Melissa is correct: She carries a great deal of tension in her shoulders and upper body. Adjusting posture and increasing awareness of her center of gravity will help her improve communication with Belle.

Remedy

At the halt I have Melissa do some small *Pelvic Rocking: Front to Back* exercises in the saddle. I coach her to use her abdominal muscles, *not* her gluteal muscles, to move her pelvis in a tuck (this is hard to do in the saddle; it is best to first learn this movement off the horse). I have her feel how the weight underneath her pelvic floor changes toward her sacrum as her pelvis moves. I then have her stop when her seat bones are underneath her. This takes the excessive arch out of her spine, engages her abdominal muscles, and helps her feel heavier in the saddle, with positive muscle tone around her center of gravity.

"But I feel like I'm hunched forward," claims Melissa.

Many with an extended posture feel slouched when their alignment is changed. I have her look in the mirror, and she sees how she looks more centered and less perched in the saddle.

"Okay," she says as she views her position. "Now, how do I keep this position?"

I have Melissa imagine that her abdominal muscles work like strong bungee cords attaching her ribs to her pelvis, preventing her spine from arching. A "hum" of tone from her abdominal muscles supports a more correct posture and eases shoulder tension.

Back out on the rail, Melissa begins to revert to her extended position.

I coach her to keep the bungee cords short to keep her ribs down, and to feel the weight over her pelvic floor shift back toward her sacrum.

At the posting trot Melissa begins to feel a more stable balance. However, when Belle speeds up, Melissa reverts to her extended posture and tense upper back and shoulders, and pulls on the reins. I coach her to steady Belle's trot tempo with her posting tempo and to breathe and focus on her core for balance to decrease tension in her shoulders.

Belle begins to respond to Melissa's improved posture and balance by keeping a steadier trot tempo. For some steps, Belle even begins to lower her head and reach to the bit.

Exercises: *Pelvic Rocking on Ball: Front to Back; Abdominal Curls; Bounce in Rhythm 2: Arm Swings.*

A Pretty Picture

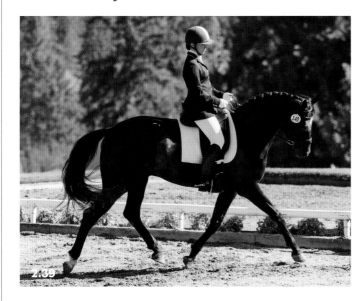

Catherine Reid on the 2006 Hanoverian gelding Skywalker HW could easily fall into an extended (arched) back position on this turn, but she keeps a correct "ribs-to-pelvis" length in the front of her body to avoid a change in her posture. Catherine notes that Skywalker can entice her to lean back at the waist if he gets sluggish in the corners and a bit heavy in the bridle, causing her to arch her back. A helpful exercise to remind her of correct alignment and avoid arching is Pelvic Rocking: Front-to-Back (done sitting in the saddle rather than on the ball) emphasizing the "Front" movement. In this way, Catherine is reminded of the correct contact with her pelvic floor in the saddle during her ride.

to be sure these muscles are helping support posture. At first, many riders will feel as if they are hunched, slouched, or flexed forward. But, by getting more support from the abdominal muscles, they will also feel more stable, which promotes suppleness in the shoulder girdle and a more elastic connection through the bridle. In the extended posture, the back muscles are doing most of the balance work, and the front of the body—the abdominal region—is too long (see fig. 2.8 C, p. 29). Accessing all of the core muscles to support posture (and balance) avoids straining the back muscles as the workload is spread over more muscle groups. Useful exercises include *Pelvic Rocking Supine; Pelvic Rocking on Ball*; and *Abdominal Curls*.

S-Shaped Posture

Some riders, especially those with a long, tall torso, ride with too much curve in the lumbar, thoracic, and cervical regions of the spine. Their back is overarched in the lumbar region, and the pelvis is tilted so that the seat bones point back. At the same time, the rider's upper back is rounded and pushed back behind the vertical, while the shoulders are rounded forward. There may also be too

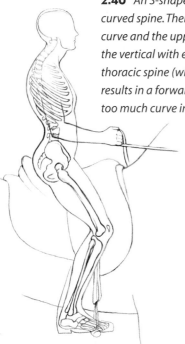

2.40 *An S-shaped posture or overly curved spine. There is excessive lumbar curve and the upper back is behind the vertical with excessive curve in the thoracic spine (where the ribs attach). This results in a forward-thrusting head with too much curve in the cervical spine.*

much curve in the neck so that the chin juts forward (fig. 2. 40). The long torso is challenging to support and keep stable on horseback. For these riders, the problem often starts with a tendency to position the upper body behind the vertical by hinging at the waist with shoulders rounded forward. The other regions of the spine, the low back and the neck, compensate for this off-balanced position with increased curvature.

These riders often find it difficult to ride comfortably, and some complain of back pain. They often look unstable and too "movable" in their midsection, as their postural support is unsteady and unbalanced. The forward-positioned chin and tight shoulders can cause a head bob, particularly noticeable at sitting trot. It is very challenging to address all of the regions of the spine at once, but without doing so, stability and balance are precarious.

Remedy

For this postural issue, I first adjust the pelvis so that the seat bones point down. This requires abdominal-muscle activation, bringing the pubic bone

A Pretty Picture

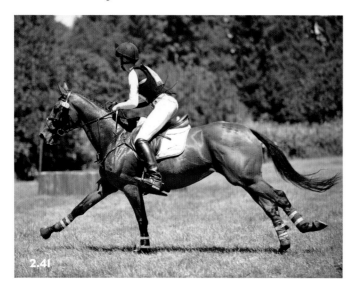

2.41

The long torso of Patience O'Neal is admirably held in correct posture while galloping cross-country on her 2003 Thoroughbred mare True Avenue (aka "Avi"). The dynamic state of galloping challenges the strongest of riders. This young rider could easily slump into an unstable and movable S-shape spine alignment compromising her balance and communication with Avi. But with her stable position, she is able to steady and prepare Avi for the next jump on the course. If you struggle keeping a stable alignment while galloping—or at any gait—practice the integrating core exercises: Plank on Mat: Knees; Plank on Mat: Feet; Plank on Ball; Quadruped: Single; and Quadruped: Diagonal for improved postural support.

Correcting S-Shaped Posture

In A, Anne Appleby demonstrates an extreme "S" posture on her 1998 Hanoverian FEI gelding Lottery TF. Note that Anne's spine has too much curve in the lumbar region, the thoracic region, as well as the cervical spine (neck). It is a challenge for any rider with such a long torso to have sufficient core-muscle awareness and tone to support this body type in neutral spine alignment, considering all the movement-energy input from a moving horse. Many riders with a similar body type risk adopting this posture.

In B, Anne corrects this posture by first bringing her seat bones more underneath her body (shortening the front of her body, decreasing the extension, or arch, in her lumbar spine) and then bringing her shoulder blades together and pressing her upper back forward (decreasing the excessive flexion, that is, the rounding of her upper back). She also stretches her neck long and is careful to keep her gaze up in front of her. She imagines the "lower plate" of her abdominal region pressing back, and her "upper plate" of her shoulder region pressing forward to support this more upright posture. Off-horse exercises that are helpful to develop the needed awareness and muscle tone to maintain neutral spine in a rider with a long torso include: *Spine Extension: Scarecrow; Spine Extension on Mat; Pelvic Rocking: Front to Back; Plank on Mat: Knees* or *Plank on Mat: Feet.*

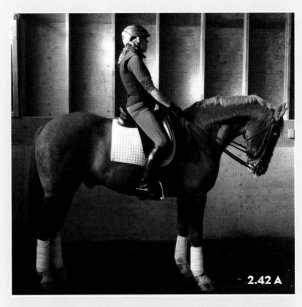

2.42 A

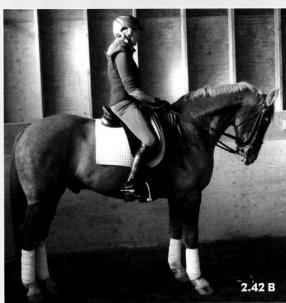

2.42 B

Consequences of S-Shaped Posture
Causes unstable balance
Puts rider behind the motion, "leaning" on the reins
Extends (arches) lumbar spine, leaving it unsupported and risking strain
Extends cervical spine, leaving it unsupported and risking strain
Leads to a head bob due to the associated tight shoulder girdle
Precludes self-carriage in both horse and rider as they are "holding each other up" through the bridle

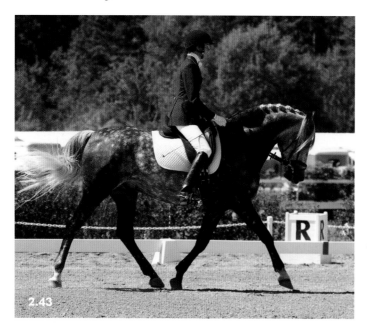

2.43

Garyn Heidemann has a long torso, and risks falling into an "S" posture. Here on the 2003 Friesian/Arab cross gelding Gabriel (owned by Kelly O'Toole) she is nicely upright in her position. Garyn notes that Gabriel is usually light in the bridle, but he can be spooky. She is always working to keep him engaged in the work by riding figures and transitions. When this gelding gets distracted, Garyn finds his large neck can be a physical challenge to keep under control without disruption of her posture. Spine Extension: Scarecrow and Plank on Mat: Knees or Plank on Mat: Feet are useful exercises for Garyn to support her correct alignment every step of the ride.

RIDER'S CHALLENGE

The S-Shaped Posture

Jennifer, an experienced advanced rider, contacts me for a position consultation.

"I dislike watching my videotapes from horse shows. I don't like the lack of elegance in my position. Plus, my back is sometimes sore after riding," she explains.

Jennifer rides a five-year-old gelding, Jupiter, a Thoroughbred/Percheron cross. Jennifer is a positive leader for the young horse, but he tends to be heavy on his forehand, barreling around the arena.

I watch Jennifer as she rides in a forward posting trot, sitting trot, and canter. Jennifer has a slight build, long legs, and a long torso. It is challenging to maintain this long spine in a stable neutral position, especially in the context of a heavy horse. Jupiter's balance difficulties have affected Jennifer's posture and effectiveness:

She has adopted a classic S-shaped position that has her upper body rounded back behind the vertical, with too much arch in her lumbar spine. Further, to counterbalance her backward-leaning upper body, her chin juts out. The backward leaning and rounded upper body is likely in response to Jupiter's being on the forehand: Jennifer uses her body weight against his leaning, supporting a mutual "hold each other up" situation. The resulting tightness of her shoulder girdle causes a head bob visible in the sitting trot. As well, excessive lumbar spine movement makes her appear unstable in the sitting trot, rather than elegant and balanced. This excess movement of the lumbar spine could be causing her back soreness.

Remedy

At the halt, I give Jennifer my "planes" images: I have her imagine that the back of her upper body forms one of the pelvis closer to the sternum of the rib cage. However, if that is the only correction, the rider remains rounded forward in the upper back and shoulders, with continued stress at the neck. So, at the same time as activating the abdominal muscles, the upper back muscles must also engage to bring the thoracic spine into a straighter alignment, lift the sternum, and bring the shoulders back and down. Finally, to straighten the cervical spine, the rider needs to stretch upward through the back of the neck, as if "on the bit."

To help hold the position in the body, I suggest that the rider imagines that the upper back is one plane, and the abdominal region is another. These two planes are parallel to each other but are separated by the width of the rider's body. To achieve improved spine alignment and stability, both planes are drawn toward the center of the body (fig. 2.44). This dynamic activity lengthens the spine and takes the excess curvature out of the lumbar and thoracic spines. The neck position then often corrects itself or is relatively easy to reposition (see figs. 2.42 A & B, p. 63).

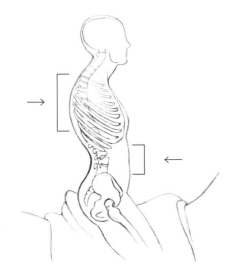

2.44 *Feel a plane of the upper back and a plane in the lower abdomen; when these planes come toward the middle of the body, excess curves are removed and the spine is supported in better alignment.*

plane. The front of her lower body, or her abdominal region, forms another plane. To promote stability of her long torso, I have her picture the two planes coming close together in the middle of her body. This activates the spine extensors in her upper back to support a more upright, less-rounded upper back position, as well as the abdominal muscles, to support a less-arched lumbar spine. As a final cue, I have her stretch the back of her neck long, imagining that she is "on the bit."

These three maneuvers take out the excessive curves in her lumbar, thoracic, and cervical spine regions, and activate postural muscles to preserve this alignment despite Jupiter's pulling. To test her ability to keep this alignment, I stand in front of Jupiter's chest, hold on to the reins, and pull against Jennifer's body and posture. By keeping her planes coming together in the middle of her body, she maintains proper posture despite the load.

Jennifer struggles to preserve this new alignment in sitting trot. I encourage her to do circles or transitions to help Jupiter's balance, rather than slip into her usual holding pattern. With improved awareness of how Jupiter coaxes her into holding him up, she becomes more particular about him maintaining his own balance, and rides with improved precision and higher standards.

Jennifer's sliding into her "S" posture demonstrates how horses can change you! Setting high posture and alignment standards for yourself makes you a better horse trainer: In a position of clear and stable balance, you can more readily detect and correct the horse's problem.

Exercises: *Pelvic Rocking Supine; Spine Extension: Scarecrow; Plank on Ball; Plank on Mat: Knees; Plank on Mat: Feet.*

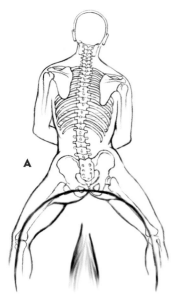

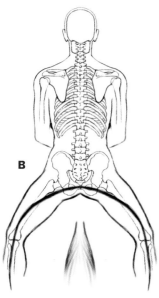

2.45 A & B *In A, the rider shows a lateral imbalance: the right side is shortened; the weight is shifted to the left; the right shoulder is low; the left shoulder is high. This is often accompanied by a pulling up and in of the right hip-joint muscles, and loss of the stirrup on this short side. In B, the rider has good lateral balance.*

The *Plank on Ball* and *Plank on Mat* exercises discussed earlier in this chapter, when done correctly, will strengthen the muscles that pull the two body planes together in the middle. However, it is easy to perform these exercises incorrectly and exaggerate the excess curves. Prepare carefully for them and think "shoulders back and down, and abdominal muscles inward" at the same time. If this results in pain or straining, stop and seek input. *Spine Extension: Scarecrow* also facilitates support of the thoracic spine.

Lateral Postural Imbalance

Imbalance of the postural muscles can interfere with side-to-side, or lateral, symmetry (figs. 2.45 A & B). I am amazed at how often this type of imbalance occurs in riders: I have seen it in over 80 percent of the riders I have worked with, from beginning to advanced. Positive changes in rider lateral balance can bring remarkable improvements in horse-and-rider function, balance, and harmony.

Seemingly small adjustments in how you support your body can improve your horse's way of going and his response to aids. It is a rider-position issue, more than any other, where your horse's way of going gives you immediate feedback. The horse's improvement quickly informs you that you've made positive changes in your position even though they are difficult to do, argue with your habits, and do not feel normal!

No one is perfectly symmetric, and just like our horses, most of us have a tendency to be stronger on one side than the other. The muscles on the strong side of the body are shorter and will tend to pull the pelvis and thighbone up off the saddle, causing an inward curve of that side of the body. This shifts weight onto the pelvis and seat bone of the weaker, longer side. This is usually accompanied by a slight spinal rotation toward the stronger side. Sometimes, but not always, this asymmetry is related to handedness—that is, a right-handed rider will tend to have a stronger right side of the body: The right side is short and contracted, and weight is shifted onto the left seat bone; and the right arm and leg are dominant. While you might overcome and correct these

Correcting Lateral Postural Imbalance

In A, Kirsten Miller demonstrates lateral imbalance on her 1998 Norwegian Fjord mare Bergen Saundra. Kirsten sits heavily to the left. You can see how her right side is short and her left side is long. She is a "right-sided" rider, that is, her body is short and contracted on her right side, which causes her weight to shift to the left.

To correct this posture, in B, Kirsten lifts up the left side of her pelvis, taking weight off the heavy left side. This restores balance over her seat bones. *Pelvic Rocking: Side to Side, Side Planks: Knees,* and *Side Planks: Feet* are great exercises for Kirsten to develop awareness and control of her core muscles to preserve lateral balance in the saddle.

Consequences of Lateral Postural Imbalance
Makes straightness of the horse very difficult
Risks giving horse conflicting aids
Makes balance in bending lines and lateral movements very difficult
Creates or contributes to lateral imbalance in the horse

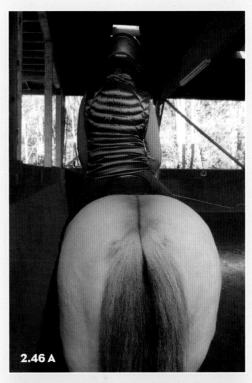

2.46 A

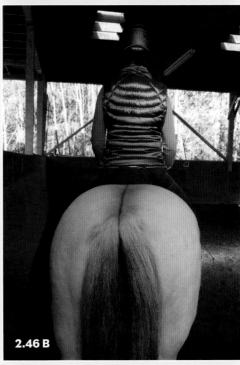

2.46 B

imbalances during daily activity without much problem, they become much more pronounced in the precarious and unpredictable environment of riding.

This right-to-left asymmetry is sometimes described as "collapsing," that is, the rider is collapsing on the short, strong side. In some ways, it looks like the rider is falling over toward the short side. This is not the best way to describe the problem, however, because "collapsing" implies being passive or soft. This imbalance is anything but passive or soft. The short side is the overactive, strong, and contracted side; the long, weighted side is the side that is not doing its part to support position, symmetry, and balance.

Sometimes an instructor might guide a rider to "push weight onto" or "sit down on" the lifted side of the pelvis or seat bone. But, since muscles only shorten and pull to move bones, there is no way to push the lifted seat bone down onto the saddle.

Remedy

Lateral asymmetry is best corrected by thinking of engaging the trunk muscles of the longer, weaker side and lifting weight off the heavily weighted side of the pelvis (see figs. 2.46 A & B). This leads to a more balanced use of the muscles of the sides of the trunk and equalizes the weight distribution over the seat bones and pelvic floor in the saddle. It takes great energy and focus to change this habitual support pattern. Improving lateral balance starts with awareness and muscle coordination.

Since lateral imbalances are so engrained in our daily movement patterns, I strongly advise off-horse movements and exercises to help you understand your tendencies and learn what it feels like to be laterally centered. I don't know if it is possible to be completely symmetrical, but we can try!

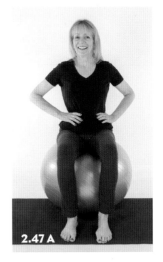

2.47 A

EXERCISES for Symmetry and Lateral Balance

As with any postural abnormality, addressing the issue starts with awareness. The first of this next exercise series is a "regular" in my RiderPilates classes. If you can master a fairly symmetrical *Pelvic Rocking on Ball: Side to Side*, you are well on your way to feeling symmetry in your body, perceiving when lateral balance fails, and having a tool to correct the imbalance. As well, *Spine Twist* teaches you how to be laterally balanced while turning. Finally, *Side Planks* improves strength in the muscles of the waist used for lateral balance.

Pelvic Rocking on Ball: Side to Side
Use your back and abdominal muscles to adjust the lateral position of the pelvis.

1 Sit on an exercise ball in neutral alignment, feet in front of you, flat on the floor.

2 Place your hands on your waist: This helps you feel the trunk muscles engage during the exercise (fig. 2.47 A).

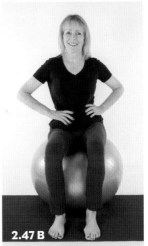

2.47 B

3 Lift up the left side of your pelvis, engaging the trunk muscles on that side, while sinking weight onto your right seat bone (fig. 2.47 B). Imagine that you are shortening the distance between your armpit and pelvis on your left side.

4 Come back to the start position, and repeat on your right side (fig. 2.47 C). Do 8 to 10 swings side to side.

Most riders have one side for which this exercise is straightforward (the strong side), and one side for which it is not (the weaker side). Feel what happens on the easier side. Try to duplicate this on the other side. Be careful not to shift your shoulders to the side or twist your body. The motion is a small side-to-side movement of your pelvis by the trunk muscles, like a swinging pendulum. Try not to use your gluteal muscles or other leg muscles to move your pelvis. Keep your feet flat on the floor.

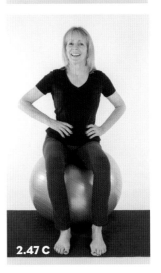

2.47 C

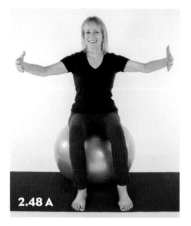

2.48 A

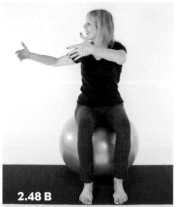

2.48 B

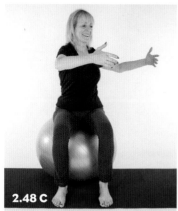

2.48 C

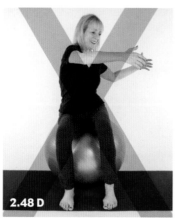

2.48 D

Spine Twist on Ball

Improves awareness of lateral balance while turning.

1 Sit upright on an exercise ball, feet on the floor, hip-joint width apart.

2 Lift up your arms and hold them in a big circle out in front of you, as if you were holding a huge ball (fig. 2.48 A).

3 Take an easy inhale breath, and on the exhale breath, rotate your upper body (rib cage, shoulders, and head) to the right (fig. 2.48 B). Then inhale back to center and exhale while you rotate your upper body to the left (fig. 2.48 C) and inhale back to center.

4 Repeat this twist or rotation of your spine 6 to 8 times each direction.

Keep your seat bones equally weighted during this exercise. It is tempting to sink onto your seat bone on the side opposite the direction of the twist (2.48 D). If you do find yourself sinking, keep that seat bone lifted so that your weight stays in the middle of the ball throughout the movement (using the tools taught in *Pelvic Rocking on Ball: Side to Side*). Keep your upper body moving as one unit, so your arms do not move more than your torso. Let your gaze follow the movement.

This exercise helps you learn that you can move your upper body independently from your lower body, and that you can turn your upper body without an obligatory shift in weight. This allows you, while riding your horse on a circle, to keep your shoulders in line with your horse's shoulders, and at the same time, keep your weight balanced over your horse's back.

Side Plank on Mat: Knees

Side Planks strengthen the muscles in your waist, developing a tool for lateral balance.

1 Lie on your left side with your left elbow in line under your left armpit; your upper arm bone should be perpendicular to the floor.

2 Stack one leg on top of the other, positioned so that they are in line with the rest of your body, with your hip joints straight. Bend your knees so the lower legs are behind you.

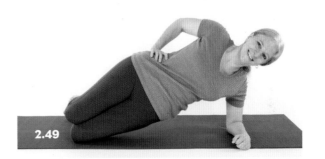

3 Place your right hand on your waist.

4 From the muscles of your left waist, lift yourself up onto your left elbow and your left knee by engaging the core muscles of your left torso (fig. 2.49). Keep your body lifted from the middle, as if a rope were around your midsection, pulling you up to the ceiling.

5 Hold the position for 15 to 30 seconds. Repeat on the right side.

Be careful that you do not push away from your elbow; your upper arm should stay perpendicular to the floor. Too much angle at the shoulder is straining.

Side Plank on Mat: Feet
A much more challenging version of *Side Plank*.

1 Lie on your left side, with your left elbow in line under your left armpit.

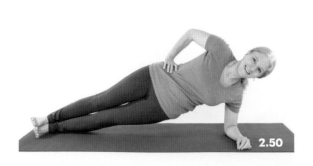

2 Stack one leg on top of the other, positioned so that they are in line with the rest of your body with your knee and hip joints straight.

3 Place your right hand on your waist.

4 From the muscles of your left waist, lift yourself up onto your left elbow and your left foot by engaging the core muscles of your left torso (fig. 2. 50). If this is too challenging, place one foot in front of the other. Keep your body lifted from the middle, as if a rope were around your midsection pulling you up to the ceiling.

5 Hold the position for 15 to 30 seconds. Repeat on the right side.

Be careful that you do not push away from your elbow; your upper arm should stay perpendicular to the floor. Too much angle at the shoulder is straining.

Lateral Imbalance Effects on Rider Function

Lateral imbalances affect horse-and-rider function in both overt and subtle ways. These are some manifestations of lateral imbalance that I have observed (a given rider may have one or more). I call a "right-sided" rider one that is short and contracted on her right side and sits heavily on the left seat bone; a "left-sided" rider is short and contracted on her left side and sits heavily on the right seat bone. (Note to instructors: To gain more information about the horse and rider's lateral balance, watch your client from the outside of their riding path so you can see both sides of the rider.)

The Right-Sided Rider:

• Sits too far to the left when tracking to the right, causing the horse to fall out on the left shoulder.

• Sits to the left when tracking left, so the horse resists left bend or falls in on the circle left.

• Rotates her upper body to the right, tracking both to the right and to the left.

• Tends to overuse the right arm and rein regardless of direction of travel; the horse's neck is over-bent going to the right; the horse's neck is restricted and either counter-bent or not allowed to bend left when tracking left.

• Tightens her right leg, with the right knee pulled up and into the knee roll of the saddle. The right leg has to grip to prevent her from falling farther off to the left side. As a result, the rider tends to lose the right stirrup and has a hard time controlling the right leg.

• Heavily weights the left stirrup, sometimes pressing the leg forward. The left leg may lack function because it is stuck carrying excess weight.

• Has a right shoulder that is lower than the left shoulder.

• Tilts her head to the right.

The Left-Sided Rider:

• Sits too far to the right when tracking to the left, causing the horse to fall out on the right shoulder.

• Sits to the right when tracking right, so the horse resists the right bend or falls in on the circle right.

• Rotates her upper body to the left, tracking both to the right and to the left.

- Tends to overuse the left arm and rein regardless of direction of travel; the horse's neck is over-bent going to the left; the horse's neck is restricted and either counter-bent or not allowed to bend right when tracking right.

- Tightens her left leg, with the left knee pulled up and into the knee roll of the saddle. The left leg has to grip to prevent her from falling farther off to the right side. As a result, the rider tends to lose the left stirrup and has a hard time controlling the function of the left leg.

- Heavily weights the right stirrup, sometimes pressing the leg forward. The right leg may lack function because it is stuck carrying excess weight.

- Has a left shoulder that is lower than the right shoulder.

- Tilts her head to the left.

Lateral Imbalance Effects on Movement

A lateral imbalance can make a simple problem worse. Imagine a *right-sided rider* sitting left while *tracking right*, and the horse is falling out the left shoulder. The rider may respond by adding more inside rein, which will over-bend the horse's neck, causing the horse to fall even more to the left. The unsuspecting rider reacts by pulling more on the right rein, further activating her right side and shifting her weight farther to the left; the horse falls more out on the left shoulder and farther away from the desired direction of travel. This unbalanced picture can be dysfunctional enough to disturb the horse's rhythm or send the pair into the arena wall.

When *tracking left*, the right-sided rider tends to sit with weight shifted to the left, or to the inside of a circle. Her body is also rotated to the right, so her shoulders are not aligned with the horse's shoulders. On a left circle, the horse tends to fall in on the left shoulder. The rider may try to "hold up" the horse's left shoulder with the left (inside) rein or may try to rebalance through the right (outside) rein. The right rein may already be restricted by the rider's dominant right side and arm. This further unbalances the horse onto the left shoulder and gives the horse a mixed message ("go left" with the left rein; "don't go left" with the right rein). It is hard for the rider to access her left leg to encourage left bend as her balance is unsteady, her left leg is heavily weighted, and the left leg and side tend to be the lazy side anyway.

Lateral imbalance can also complicate *lateral* movements. For example, the leg-yield can be quite different depending upon direction. I'm going to give examples for a right-sided rider, however, read it vice versa for the left-sided rider.

For a *right*-sided rider, the leg-yield going to the left may feel relatively easy because the rider already sits in that direction However, the quality of the movement likely suffers because the horse is not in balance: He tends to fall onto the left shoulder rather than carrying with the right hind leg.

The leg-yield to the *right* can be challenging because the rider's weight is to the left but her aids are trying say "go to the right." This can lead to confusion and resistance in the horse, and the "need" for stronger and stronger aids from the rider (fig. 2.51).

Remedy

Adapting some of my simple ball exercises to the saddle can improve lateral symmetry. *Pelvic Rocking: Side to Side* in the saddle will help you access the torso muscles on the long, less-strong side of your body and introduce the feeling of being truly in the middle of the saddle. Again, the pelvic floor reference is helpful to guide you to feel that it is possible to keep fairly even weight over both right and left seat bones when your pelvis is centered in the saddle from balanced-torso muscle function. When practicing this exercise in the saddle, however, be sure to use the muscles of your torso (deep abdominal and back muscles), not the muscles of your legs (your gluteal muscles and/or

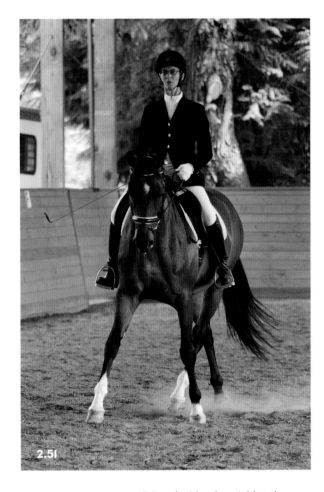

2.51

DG and I ride a leg-yield to the right. I am a "right-sided" rider so I struggle to keep my weight from falling left as I use my left leg in this leg-yield. I keep my left waist supported to avoid falling leftward so I can stay in the middle of the saddle. I do a few Pelvic Rocking: Side to Side movements in the saddle at the beginning of each ride to clarify what it feels like to sit in the center of the saddle.

your hip flexors), to adjust pelvic position. If your leg muscles move your pelvis, they become involved in posture and postural support and are not available for leg aids. It is very important for you to make adjustments in your posture or pelvic position using your torso muscles.

The *Spine Twist* exercise, done in a small range of motion in the saddle, teaches you that it is possible to turn your upper body a little bit in both directions without disturbing the weight over your pelvic floor. You learn the skill of turning your upper body either right or left and are thus able to keep your shoulders aligned with your horse's shoulders, regardless of direction of travel, without disturbing balance.

RIDER'S CHALLENGE ||||||||||||||||||||||||||||||||||||||||||||||||||||||||||||||||||||||||||||||||||||||||||||||||||||||||||||

Lateral Balance

Christina trots up on her attractive grey Oldenburg gelding, Max. She is smartly turned out and quite earnest in her attitude.

"I need for him to be more responsive to my aids," she says.

I watch the two of them for a few minutes. Christina has a fairly short torso with proper spine alignment front to back. As she executes a left turn at the posting trot, however, she falls off to the right and over-bends Max's neck to the left. He resists and tosses his head; Christina responds by more pulling on the left rein and a kick with her left leg. They continue around the left turn with Max in a flat, irregular trot rhythm, resisting the left rein and falling to the right.

On the right rein, Christina turns her body to the left and crosses her left (outside) hand over Max's neck to the right to get Max to turn right. He resists and tosses his counter-bent neck, his trot again losing a regular rhythm.

Christina's struggles with lateral balance contribute to the communication difficulties she experiences with Max. She is a left-sided rider—that is, short and contracted on her left side, with her weight shifted to the right, regardless of direction of travel.

Remedy

I have Christina do the *Pelvic Rocking: Side to Side* and *Spine Twist* exercises in the saddle to help her become aware of her unbalanced weight distribution over her pelvic floor. It is very difficult for her to accomplish lifting the right side of her pelvis with the muscles of her right waist region, and she resorts to lifting her right shoulder, twisting her body, and lifting her right leg. With some persistence, she is able to connect to the muscles of her right torso and improve her balance over her pelvic floor.

I point out that just like our horses, our bodies have their own "evasions" and assure Christina that she is not alone with this balance challenge. Day-to-day living results in right-left asymmetries in our body. When we put ourselves in the precarious and unpredictable position of being on horseback, these habits come in loud and strong. It takes a huge conscious effort to change them. Correcting this asymmetry starts with awareness. Then we try to replace the ingrained habits

Your "Elbow Spur"

If you struggle with lateral balance, you may find it helpful to imagine a small spur (like the one you may wear on your boot) on the inside of the elbow of your long, heavily weighted side (for the *right*-sided rider, this is the left side; for the *left*-sided rider, the right). The job of this "elbow spur" is to keep the long side tucked in and engaged, doing its part to help stabilize alignment and balance.

Imagine you are a right-sided rider. When *tracking right*, you need to prevent your weight from falling too far to the left. Your left "elbow spur" keeps your torso going a bit to the right and prevents it from bowing out to the left.

with more productive stabilizing strategies. Our horses quickly reward us when our alignment improves.

I have Christina track right and think of her body bending right in the same way she wants her horse to bend right. By rotating her upper body to the right and engaging her right waist, Christina keeps her shoulders aligned with Max's shoulders, and reduces her excessive weight on her right seat bone. It is difficult for her to make these changes, but each time she convinces her body to rotate right and be more centered, she is able to release her overly tight grip on the left (outside) rein, Max's neck stretches toward the bit, and his trot gains cadence.

"I can't believe the change in his trot with what feels like such a tiny change in my body!" she exclaims.

To the left, Christina has a much more difficult time accessing the right side of her body to keep herself in lateral balance. She persists in over-rotating her body to the left and hanging on the left rein while the two of them fall to the right.

I have Christina rotate her upper body a bit right, or to the outside, to correct her excessive leftward rotation. I have her think of steering Max's shoulders: to turn him

left, bring his right shoulder to the left. I have her lift her weight off her right pelvis to bring Max to the left, by engaging the muscles of her right waist. Two images help her: a rope around her waist pulling her to the center of the circle (activating her right waist muscles) and bringing her right side to the left; and installing a "spur" on her right elbow that prevents her body from falling too far right.

Christina struggles with her balance to the left, but when she is able to shift her weight from off the right seat bone onto the middle of her pelvis, she becomes more elastic in the contact through the left rein, Max is straighter, and again, he reaches for the bit with improved cadence.

"My brain is exhausted," she says at the end of the ride. "But Max was better!"

This lateral-balance issue is such a challenge to work on because our movement habits can be very ingrained. Max rewarded Christina for her efforts—there is no better feedback than that!

Exercises for Christina: *Pelvic Rocking on Ball: Side to Side; Spine Twist on Ball; Side Plank on Mat: Knees and Feet.*

It may also help to think of steering your horse's withers by bringing the left side of your body toward the right. This helps keep weight appropriately on your right seat bone. You must be careful to not over-bend the horse's neck to accomplish the turn; instead, bring the outside of your horse to the right with your torso and, sometimes, with your left upper thigh.

Again, imagine you are a right-sided rider. When *tracking left*, you must make a conscious effort to turn your shoulders to the left and rotate your body a bit to the left; in essence, you, like your horse, need to bend left. This is not a natural way of positioning yourself, but in doing so, your weight will be more centered, and your left leg will be able to support your horse's bend. Rotating your torso left with the horse's shoulders also guides you to allow the left bend of the horse's neck through the right (outside) rein. Your left "elbow spur" keeps up its job of activating your left torso, as well.

When you achieve improved balance going right and then left, changes of direction can be introduced through, for example, a figure eight. This movement helps you hone in on finding and staying in the middle of the saddle regardless of direction of travel. With improved balance, your horse's way of going will dramatically improve, and resistances and evasions will lessen.

Certainly the horse's balance and asymmetries play a role in the scenarios I've described, but since you are the cognitive, problem-solving member of the partnership, you must recognize your role in this lateral (or any other!) balance problem. When you have found stability and balance in the middle of the saddle, you can then influence your horse and help him balance more efficiently. You are able to quickly feel if your horse falls one way or the other and can help your horse regain balance, rather than make it worse. You become more perceptive and effective.

To remind you, lateral postural imbalances are hard to address when your front-to-back balance is unstable. When I train riders, I do not focus on lateral balance until there is an understanding of the balance between the muscles of the front and the back of the body.

Lateral asymmetry can get worse when working on a new movement or figure. The effort devoted to learning the new material prompts the brain to return to its habitual balance patterns. The need for strong arm or leg aids can also challenge your stability to the point that this postural imbalance becomes more pronounced. As in horse training, I advise riders to take a step back when the balance gets worse, correct it, regroup, and try again. And don't forget to breathe!

Unbalanced "X" Posture

A final postural problem, the *unbalanced "X" posture*, is very challenging to address. It is one where the rider has a more complicated asymmetry that causes her weight at the pelvis to go one direction and her upper body to go the other. Straightness for the horse is thus very challenging.

Imagine your torso as a rectangle. Draw a line from your right shoulder to your left pelvis, and your left shoulder to your right pelvis. You have drawn an "X" on your torso. Most people have equal arms of this "X." Some, however, particularly those with scoliosis, or abnormal lateral curvature of the spine, have one arm of the "X" longer than the other (fig. 2.52). At times, I have seen this compensation in riders with a lateral imbalance problem (see p. 66). Rather than truly addressing the unbalanced weight over both seat bones, the crafty body of some riders will adjust by simply shifting the mobile upper body and shoulders to the less-weighted side of the body. The pelvis remains too far off to one side, with the shoulders too far to the other. This takes one problem and creates two!

Remedy

This is a challenging balance strategy to correct, particularly if an underlying abnormal spine curvature exists. But, if you have this issue, you can begin to feel straighter with this imagery: Let's say that your "X" imbalance has your right-shoulder-to-left-pelvis distance longer than your left-shoulder-to-right-pelvis distance. To be straight, you need to shift your rib cage to the left and shift your pelvis to the right. You can begin to feel this by putting your right hand under your right armpit and pressing to the center of your body. At the same time, put your left hand on the left side of your pelvis and press it toward

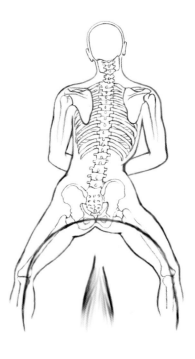

2.52 *Unbalanced "X" posture. The distance between the right shoulder and left pelvis is longer than the distance between the left shoulder and right pelvis. This imbalance can be corrected by imagining a plane under the right armpit pressing to the center of the body, and a plane at the left pelvis pressing to the center of the body.*

the center of your body. These movements bring the two arms of your torso "X" closer to symmetry. Your torso becomes more like a rectangle than a slanted parallelogram. As well, keeping your elbows close by the sides of your rib cage can help you recognize when your rib cage tends to shift to one side or the other—your arms define a corridor for your body.

Other helpful exercises include *Pelvic Rocking on Ball: Side to Side; Spine Twist on Ball; Plank on Mat: Knees and Feet; Plank on Ball; Side Plank on Mat: Knees and Feet;* and *Quadruped: Single and Diagonal.*

Seeking and maintaining proper posture improves your awareness of your horse's imbalances. Fine-tuning your balance helps you quickly recognize when your horse's issues threaten to change your body position. Allowing your horse's movement and evasions to change your posture makes you a less effective rider. Defining and maintaining correct posture makes you a clear leader, able to set precise standards for you and your horse.

With a secure posture, the goals of body control—awareness and control of your *legs* and *arms*—become much more reasonable and doable. Next, I'll talk about these body parts.

MY CHALLENGE |||||||||||||||||||||||||||||||||||||||||||||||||||||||||||||||||||||||||||||||||||||||||||||||||||||||||||||||||||||||

Flexed Posture

I have a tendency toward a flexed (rounded or C-shaped) posture (see p. 54). The function (or dysfunction) of my shoulder girdle and legs contributed to this posture. It took me some time to understand it. Sure, I got a lot of cues to "bring your shoulders back" while I was riding, but the changes I'd try to make rarely lasted because I didn't have a clear and useful tool to support better posture. It wasn't just about my arms. And, what's more, my temperament put me squarely in the "intense" category; in the saddle this translated into my focusing too much on what was happening within my line of sight and not feeling the whole horse.

So in addition to rounded shoulders and a tucked pelvis, my gaze tended downward, all feeding into spine flexion (C-shaped posture).

Correcting my flexed posture, of course, required me to engage (and trust) my back muscles to support a correct, upright posture. I had to be careful, however, for if I overused my back muscles, my back would hurt. Like so many position problems, the remedy was correct balance. I had to find the correct balance of tone between my abdominal muscles and back muscles. This improved my posture in the saddle, and my shoulder and leg muscles were less likely to interfere with my posture. I also strongly believe that finding core muscle balance has helped me continue riding with little or no back pain.

About Your Body: **Back Pain**

It is estimated that 85 percent of us will experience back pain at some time in our lives, and for over half, it will recur. Back pain is the second most common reason for individuals to see their primary care doctor. It contributes to health care costs both directly (the money you spend to get health care for your back) and indirectly (lost time and productivity at work). As well, back pain diminishes quality of life. Back pain is common in riders, especially those who have ridden for many years. Other risk factors for back pain include: smoking; depression; stress; a job that requires heavy lifting, twisting, and bending; or one that is sedentary.

The majority of back pain stems from damage to either the intervertebral discs or the joints between adjacent vertebrae (called zygoapophyseal joints, also known as facet joints—see fig 2.3).

As discussed in the beginning of this chapter, the design of the spine allows for a wide range of movement of your torso. However, prolonged or excessive rotation, flexion (forward bending), or extension (arching) puts added strain on the discs and joints. The intervertebral discs are particularly at risk for disruption if flexion is combined with rotation. This strains the connective tissue fibers that contain the

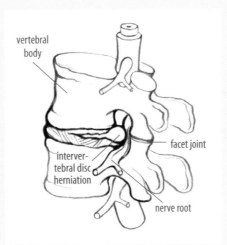

2.53 *Illustration of a herniated disc, causing compression and pain on an adjacent nerve.*

shock-absorbing disc material between each vertebra. Bulging or herniated discs, with painful pressure on adjacent nerves, can result (fig. 2.53). In addition, excessive extension places the facet joints under extra strain (see p. 82).

Correct posture, postural support, and body mechanics are key components to preventing excessive strain on the spine. Develop awareness and connection to your muscles of postural support to minimize the chance of injury. Try to maintain neutral spine alignment throughout your day. If you sit in front of a computer at work, find a way to keep good posture during that time.

Postural Issues Cause Back Pain

I meet Susan, a very experienced dressage rider and instructor, at a new clinic site. Unlike many, she does not come with a list of problems. When I ask how I can help her, she replies, "Oh I have issues, and I'm sure you'll see them."

Susan proceeds to ride her Prix St. Georges gelding, Capri, on both reins in walk, trot, and canter before moving into trot and canter lateral work. I am daunted by Susan's breadth of experience—she has trained many horses and riders to Grand Prix. How could I help her?

I start with the basic Rider Fundamentals, and find two issues in Susan's posture. First, Susan rides in a mildly extended (arched) posture with her upper body slightly in front of the vertical. The spine extension (arching) increases during down transitions, when she leans back with just her upper body.

The second postural issue is a tendency for Susan to sit with more weight on her right seat bone. She is a left-sided rider. She is short on her left side, long on her right side, and her right shoulder is usually carried higher and more forward than her left shoulder.

Remedy

To correct the extended posture, I have Susan pull her abdominal muscles in to shorten the front of her body and lengthen her shortened lumbar spine. This puts her weight farther back on her pelvic floor. It is a different feeling for her, but confers a sense a security as her pelvic position is much more stable. As a result, when she then rides some medium- to collected-trot transitions, she rides them back to front with less pulling on her part, and less bracing and hollowing in her horse. From her immense library of experience, she immediately notes the difference.

Addressing the lateral balance issue is more challenging. Susan rides eight to twelve horses a day. Her current riding position has many hours of practice. It is very difficult for her to bring her right shoulder down and back, rotate her shoulders a bit right, and shorten her right side to even out her weight in the saddle. While tracking right, her body rotates left, especially when she uses her outside (left) rein to steady her horse. Being "straight" feels quite twisted and takes tremendous mental effort to maintain.

However, the effect of a more balanced lateral position is immediately clear to Susan. In her canter and trot half-passes to the right, her lateral balance issue caused her to lean heavily on her right seat bone and press too much weight into her right stirrup. When going left, she lagged behind her horse. In her working canter pirouettes to the right, her horse fell to the right rather than keeping correct bend and carrying himself to the right. The position of her right hand gives away when she sits heavily to the right, as it lifts up and across the horse's neck to the left. When Susan corrects her lateral balance issue, the change in her horse's carriage is dramatic: The withers are more lifted, the engagement is better, and he is softer in the bridle with improved cadence. While the changes in Susan's position are small, she immediately feels the difference in her horse, and smiles!

The next time I see Susan she shares information that she had withheld during our first lesson. When we first met, Susan had so much back pain at the end of her long days that she was concerned her riding and training career days were limited. Since our first lesson, she has worked diligently on her two postural issues and has been rewarded with less back pain.

Off-horse exercises for Susan: *Pelvic Rocking on Ball: Front to Back and Side to Side; Spine Twist on Ball; Abdominal Curls; Side Plank on Mat: Knees and Feet.*

A Pretty Picture

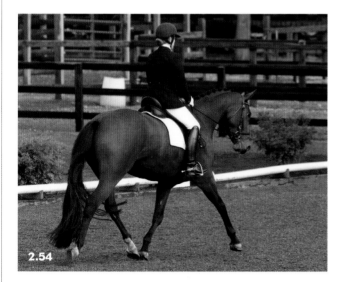

2.54

Lisa Boyer shows symmetric lateral balance on Zamora (owned by Dutch Equine Stables). Lisa praises Zamora for her quiet and generous mind, but notes that her gaits are huge! Lisa has to constantly steady herself in the middle of the saddle. If you draw a line down Lisa's back, you'll find that there is an equal amount of "Lisa" on Zamora's right and left sides. With this balance, Zamora rewards Lisa with quality movement. Pelvic Rocking: Side to Side, and Side Planks are useful exercises to help you develop lateral balance.

Riders, Keep Your Backs Healthy!

Horseback riding can contribute to back pain if good posture and body mechanics are not maintained. Fundamental to preserving back health is riding in correct posture. Recognize that spine extension (arched posture) risks straining the facet joints and that flexion (forward bending) with rotation risks damaging the intervertebral discs. Commit to riding in the best posture possible for the health of your body.

Back injuries happen off the horse, as well. Consider the lifting and "schlepping" associated with horse care—much of it can be very back unfriendly. Pay attention to body alignment and mechanics during barn chores. Avoid twisting while lifting. Keep proper spine alignment while carrying heavy objects, and lift things by bending your legs, not your spine. A good rule of thumb is to keep "your nose aligned with your toes" to prevent twisting and back strain. Move your feet to fork manure into the wheelbarrow; avoid rotating your torso. Keep heavy objects close to the front of your body. Stay focused on the task at hand so body and mind work together. Split heavy loads into several lighter loads, or get help. Use a tractor or wheelbarrow whenever possible. Use a step stool to groom a large horse so you needn't reach and twist to get at his back. Avoid fatigue! Just as with horses, this is when injuries are likely to occur.

(continued on p. 84)

(continued from p. 83)

Carefully consider the type of horse you ride. If you have back troubles, weigh the risks and benefits of working with a very green horse: The inevitable sudden movements are not ideal for your vulnerable back (while riding, leading, or longeing). Also, consider the conformation of your horse. A horse with a very round barrel may force your thighbone into a position that causes back strain. A large horse requires more lifting and reaching while grooming and tacking up. Work to improve the quality of your horse's trot before trying to sit it if it is jarring.

Barn setup can facilitate back-friendly horse care. Frequently placed hose bibs and hoses minimize the need to carry water. A hayloft allows gravity to deliver hay rather than you lifting it. Be sure walking surfaces are not slippery to minimize the risk of falls. Use a tractor that fits you to avoid reaching and straining for foot pedals and gearshifts. Make sure your horse trailer is equipped with an easily lifted ramp or a step up, and consider a motorized jack for hookup.

It may seem obvious, but remember to take good care of your body. Back health is supported by good nutrition and fitness. A good fitness program includes a mix of aerobic activity, as well as core, arm, and leg strengthening and stretching.

Finally, listen to your body. Do not ignore aches and pains. It is cheaper to hire help than to destroy your back (remember, you only have one). Depending upon your back problem, horse riding and horse care may be doable, but you must respect your body.

3 Body Control: Legs

I'll now approach the third Rider Fundamental: *Body Control—Legs*. Effective riding requires control of your legs—and arms (see chapter 4). This control is possible only when you are *focused* on your position (chapter 1) and also when the center of your body, or torso, is stable and balanced in the saddle from correct *posture,* and *postural support* from your core muscles (chapter 2). Without focus and balance from your center, your body seeks balance from your arms and/or legs, creating unwanted tension in the muscles of the hip joint, leg, and shoulder girdle. This precludes having controlled, independent, efficient, and effective leg and rein aids.

Without awareness and control, your legs fall into the role of "muscle men," causing you to use force to get what you want. Instead, you need to feel as if your legs are part of your horse's body (fig. 3.1). Your legs must move with your horse's swinging barrel or rib cage, and give appropriately

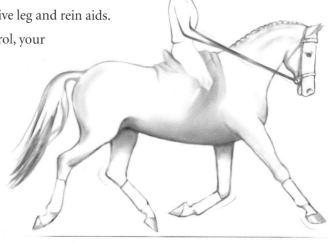

3.1 *Riding in balance allows your arms to become part of the bridle and your legs to become part of your horse's body.*

timed aids to ask for more activity, engagement, or a lateral step. You must have suitable control so you can use your right leg, left leg, or both for an aid. More advanced control allows you to use different parts of your leg for different purposes. Giving leg aids must not disrupt your balance or impair your horse's movement. A leg that is gripping to keep you from falling off cannot move with, or aid, your horse effectively. But you can only release a gripping leg when you do not need it for security, that is, when your balance is centered in your torso and supported with your engaged core muscles.

What Is the "Seat"?

You may have noticed that I do not use the term "seat" when talking about rider-position issues. I have two reasons for this. First, in my reading, I have found variable definitions for the term "seat." I do not want to risk causing misunderstanding by using a term that may mean different things to different riders. Second, there are many components to the seat in some definitions:

· Some use seat to describe your entire position and function.
· Some define seat as just your pelvis.
· Some define the seat as your pelvis and upper thigh (the body parts you sit on in the saddle).

The 2011 USDF "Glossary of Judge's Terms" offers this definition of the seat: "The control of the rider's trunk (pelvis, spine, and rib cage, with supporting musculature, not just the buttocks), producing correct dynamic influence, body function, balance, and harmony with the horse's movement (with correct influence/function within each gait and exercise)."

This definition combines some anatomy with function, but is quite broad and appears to include the hip-joint muscles ("supporting musculature") in the functional unit. I do not like to think of the pelvis and upper thigh as a single unit: I believe that awareness and control of the hip joint, connecting the thighbone to the pelvis, is crucial to good riding.

Also, riders who are directed to "use the seat" often respond by using their gluteal muscles too much. I reserve using movement of the pelvis with the gluteal muscles for advanced and sensitive horses. Before this stage, overusing the gluteal muscles results in the rider working hard with little response from the horse. This issue is demonstrated in these Rider's Challenge stories: "Overusing Gluteal Muscles" (p. 100), "Leg Aids Disrupt Posture" (p. 116) and "Pumping Gluteal Muscles at Canter" (p. 187).

In my experience, the word "intent" can replace some aspects of the term "seat." So, when you hear "drive with your seat," you can think of carrying your center of gravity in a forward direction so your body asks your horse for more ground cover, and you can back up your intent with your leg aids. For many, this is more effective than tucking your pelvis and "pushing" your horse with your gluteal muscles.

By design, in this chapter, I give basic descriptions of various leg muscle functions. It is impossible to sort out, during the busy act of riding, precisely which muscle does what, and when. When I say, for example, "Don't use your gluteal muscles," that really means use them *less*. It is not possible to have any single muscle group do nothing. My examples and illustrations show extremes to make the problems obvious. It is common for a rider to have more than one issue. But as you become aware, you can address problems and improve your effectiveness with balanced and supple leg-muscle function.

Anatomy of Legs

The leg connects to the pelvis at the hip joint (fig. 3.2) and is held in place with multiple strong ligaments. The hip joint is a "ball and socket" joint, which makes possible a great range and variety of motion at the joint. The thighbone (femur) can move forward in *flexion*, a bit back in *extension* (the hip joint does not have a big range of motion in extension), out to the side in *abduction*, toward the center of the body in *adduction*, or inward *(internal)* or outward *(external)* rotation. It is a joint that is meant to move.

The knee joint is essentially a hinge joint and moves primarily in two dimensions: *flexion* (bending the knee), and *extension* (straightening the knee). This joint is not able to allow rotation or abduction/adduction (outward/inward motion) of the lower leg to any significant degree. This will become important when I talk about how to apply leg aids.

The ankle joint is a complex joint that allows movement of the foot upward in *flexion* or downward in *extension* (or pointing the toe, also called *dorsiflexion*); the foot can also rotate inward (*inversion* or rolling onto the baby toe) and outward (*eversion* or rolling onto the great toe). Keeping the muscles of this joint supple and not locked allows the ankle to absorb movement.

In the saddle, the leg hangs from the hip joint in slight external rotation. This leg position accommodates the horse's barrel. The degree of external rotation will depend upon the rider's anatomy (a narrow pelvis leads to more

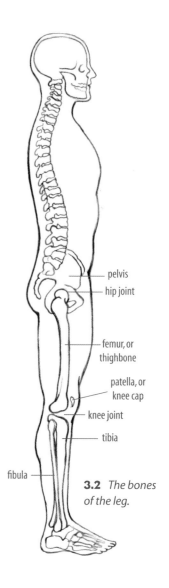

pelvis
hip joint

femur, or thighbone

patella, or knee cap

knee joint

tibia

fibula

3.2 *The bones of the leg.*

3.3 *Proper posture and leg position in the saddle results in the alignment of the shoulder, hip (pelvis), and heel.*

external rotation than a wide pelvis), the shape of the twist of the saddle, and the horse's shape (a horse with a broad back requires the rider's leg to externally rotate more than a horse that is slab-sided). This external rotation at the hip joint places the rider's knee gently against the saddle flap supported by the knee roll and places the lower leg against the horse's rib cage. It is appropriate for the rider's toe to point outward slightly, as opposed to facing straight ahead. (Because of the knee joint anatomy, pointing the toe straight ahead places rotational strain across the knee joint, causes the foot to invert at the ankle, or forces too much internal rotation at the hip joint, thus pulling the rider's knee too tightly against the saddle.)

MY CHALLENGE ||||||||||||||||||||||||||||||||||||||||||||||||||||||||||||||||||||||||||||||||||||||||||||||||||||||||||||||||||||||||||||||||||

Finding a Horse that Fits

Cautious is a word that best describes my approach to getting back in the saddle after my surgery for herniated discs in my low back. I waited a year after surgery to consider riding. And that year was full of conditioning and improving my body awareness. Finally, I was ready to find out if riding was an option for me.

I started putting feelers out for a potential mount to lease and slowly get back into riding. My criteria were strict: The horse must not have jarring gaits and must not be spooky. He must not be tall so I could avoid lifting and reaching while grooming and tacking up. I needed a reliable horse upon which I could explore strategies to keep my back supported and secure while in the saddle.

A friend told me about a 7-year-old Fjord pony mare, Solana, who needed some miles under saddle to augment her driving career. This sounded

interesting. Perhaps this breed could be a good choice for my riding rehab needs.

I met my friend at her barn one sunny afternoon. I was encouraged at how easy it was to tack up this 14.1-hand pony. We set out on a slow trail ride, and I got a feel of how Solana moved.

After about 30 minutes, my back was getting tight. Solana's back was relatively broad, requiring my thigh to externally rotate at the hip joint. This put my back in a bit of extension (arch), and caused strain. Solana's short-coupled back put a lot of swing in her rib cage as she walked, causing a great deal of movement in my pelvis and hip joint. The combination of her build and her walk put my body in a less than ideal position to move with her without strain.

So, while her size and temperament were positive features for me, Solana's body type was not.

About nine months later, after finding a more suitable mount to get me back in riding shape, I went horse shopping. Again, I was struck by how some horse shapes did not fit me well. I felt strain in my back

This balanced leg position should allow the ball of the foot to rest on the stirrup iron with a sense that just the weight of the leg sits on the stirrup, as if it is on a shelf. That is, you are neither pulling your foot off the stirrup, nor pushing weight onto the stirrup. The weight of your leg will allow your heel to rest below the level of the front of your foot, without force.

You can now add the "heel" part of the shoulder-hip (pelvis)-heel alignment of good rider position (fig. 3.3). The leg rests under your body, hanging from the balanced torso. The ideal leg position would allow you to end up standing upright on the arena surface in balance if the horse were taken out from under you.

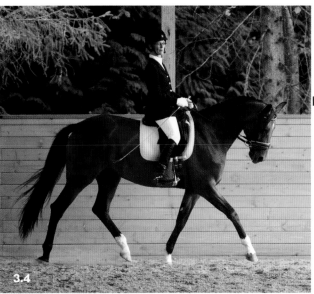

whenever I rode a horse with a broad back that put my thighbone in too much external rotation and caused my spine to arch. A more narrow-bodied horse fit me best.

I settled on Bluette, a Danish Warmblood mare cross whose dam was a Thoroughbred. Her relatively narrow conformation fit me well. Her gaits were of good quality and reasonable for me to ride. In fact, after years of training together, Bluette was my partner at Grand Prix. When horse shopping again in 2009, horse size remained an important criterion. Donner Girl, a 16-hand Oldenburg mare fit the bill (fig. 3.4).

I have worked with two clients who tell a similar story of horse size challenging comfort. Both had knee surgery for entirely different reasons. But both found that riding a horse with a round barrel placed excessive and painful strain on their knee joints: They found that applying leg aids when riding a wide-bodied horse placed unhealthy torque on the knee. However, a horse with a more narrow conformation was not a problem.

3.4

I am riding Donner Girl; "DG's" relatively small frame and size (16 hands) is a perfect fit for me. Plus, she has just the right temperament: suitably reactive so I don't usually have to use strong leg aids, but not so reactive that she is spooky and unreliable. Both of these features make her the ideal horse for me, considering my riding goals (move up the levels with her), my age (not divulging…), and my history of back issues.

If you are looking for a horse and have problems with your back, hip, or knee, don't discredit the importance of conformation in finding the right mount. Not all horse shapes suit all riders, particularly if you have a physical limitation.

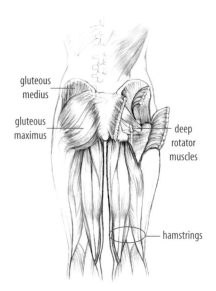

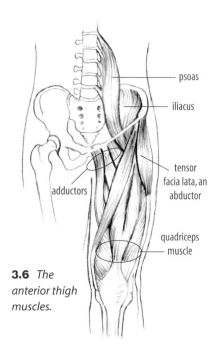

3.5 *The posterior thigh muscles.*

3.6 *The anterior thigh muscles.*

Hip Joint Muscles

A complex array of muscles connects the leg to the pelvis at the hip joint and operates the knee and ankle joints. Important hip joint muscles are shown in figures 3.5 and 3.6. Since your legs carry and propel you through the day, your leg muscles are relatively big and strong. Almost as if they have a mind of their own, your legs can demonstrate their excessive strength while you're riding—to the detriment of suppleness and efficiency. Awareness and control of these muscles is vital to allow your legs to move with your horse and give aids of appropriate pressure and timing.

Gluteal Muscles

Figure 3.5 shows the muscles of the back of the thigh. The largest muscle of the body, the *gluteus maximus,* is one of three muscles that form the gluteal muscles (or "glutes") and the contour of the buttocks. It is a strong muscle, and in conjunction with deeper muscles in the hip, extends and externally rotates the thighbone. When the thighbones are held stable, the gluteus maximus will move the pelvis in a posterior pelvic tilt (pelvic tuck).

Beneath the glutes is a collection of smaller muscles that rotate the thighbone outward. I refer to these as the *deep hip rotators.* These muscles help stabilize the rider's leg position in the saddle, working to balance inward rotation and potential gripping from the adductor muscles (see p. 101). Many riders benefit from stretching these deep rotators to facilitate freedom in the hip joint.

Hamstrings

The hamstring group of muscles forms the substance of the back of the thigh (see fig. 3.6). This group of three muscles attaches to the seat bone and to the top of the lower leg just below the knee. This muscle group extends the hip joint (it therefore assists the gluteal muscles), and flexes (bends) the knee.

The hamstrings are a powerful muscle group to access while riding, as they are the muscles that pull your lower leg against your horse's side, as well as pull your entire leg back in the saddle. This provides an efficient and specific tool for your leg aids. The degree to which your lower leg needs to move back to give the leg aid depends a bit upon your horse's sensitivity to the leg aid (which can be trained), the shape of your horse's rib cage, and the length of your leg. A sensitive horse will perceive the upper calf against his barrel, requiring little or no lower leg movement when you apply the aid. Others may require a bit more leg contact.

I believe it is better to have a brief period when your lower leg is drawn slightly back to give a leg aid than to try and keep your leg in the same position and pull your calf directly inward against your horse's side. This motion of your lower leg risks strain across your knee and sacroiliac joints. Your knee is a hinge joint, and does not easily allow this inward movement of your lower leg. As a result, you are forced to rotate your whole leg outward to accomplish this inward movement of the lower leg. This disrupts the position of both your leg and your pelvis. It is preferable to draw your lower leg back a bit, using the efficient hamstring muscle for a leg aid. Think of directing your heel toward your horse's fetlock of the opposite hind leg. This gives a line of action that activates the hamstrings and prevents your heel from coming up too much. Your leg must return to its proper position, however, after each aid.

EXERCISES for Gluteal and Hamstring Muscles

You will gain awareness of and strengthen both the *gluteal* and *hamstring* muscles in the following *Pelvic Bridge* exercises. Start with the simple exercises first; be sure you feel your glutes and hamstrings engage. As you move on to the exercises that require more balance (the *Pelvic Bridge* exercises with one leg and those using an exercise ball), organize the movement such that your core muscles stabilize balance, and the lifting of your body off the mat comes from the strong muscles of the back of your leg.

Pelvic Bridge: Simple

All of the *Pelvic Bridge* exercises strengthen your hamstrings and gluteal muscles, and activate the stabilizing muscles of your trunk.

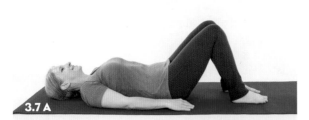 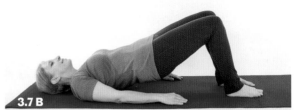

1 Lie on the floor in neutral spine alignment, knees bent, feet flat on the floor hip-joint width apart, arms by your sides (fig. 3.7 A).

2 Keeping neutral alignment, on an exhale breath, stabilize your spine then activate your gluteal and hamstring muscles to lift your pelvis and torso off the floor, until your body forms a plank from your knees to your shoulders (fig. 3.7 B).

3 Return your pelvis and torso to the mat, back to start position, as you take an inhale breath.

4 Repeat 6 to 8 times.

I have described doing this exercise in neutral spine, which makes it feel a bit like the motion of posting the trot. Be sure that the power for this exercise comes from your gluteal and hamstring muscles of the back of your leg. These muscles—not the muscles of your back or arms—lift your body off the floor.

Check that you push off from both feet equally; one leg should not do more work than the other. Keep spine alignment stable and don't let your back arch at the top of the movement; Keep your trunk muscles engaged. Don't let your knees fall apart: keep your knees aligned over your feet (placing a small ball or towel between the knees helps).

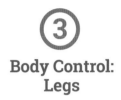

Pelvic Bridge: Single Leg

This version of *Pelvic Bridge* challenges leg strength and the ability of your torso muscles to keep your pelvis level.

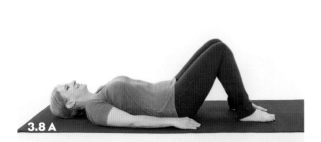 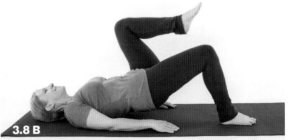

1 Lie on the floor in neutral spine alignment, knees bent, feet flat on the floor and close together in the center of your body, arms by your sides (fig. 3.8 A).

2 Lift your left knee to your chest.

3 Keeping neutral alignment, on an exhale breath, stabilize your spine then activate your gluteal and hamstring muscles on your right leg to lift your pelvis and torso off the floor, until your body forms a "plank" from your right knee to your shoulders (fig. 3.8 B).

4 Return your pelvis and torso to the mat, back to start position, as you take an inhale breath.

5 Repeat 3 to 4 times on your right leg. Repeat, lifting with just your left leg.

Try to keep the front of your pelvis level as you lift with just one leg; avoid letting one side dip down. Keep the range of motion small at first. If this exercise causes a hamstring cramp, briefly stretch your leg, and try again, focusing on balance, organization, and smooth movement. Also be sure to recruit your gluteal muscles to help with the lift. For a more challenging exercise, start with your feet seat-bone width apart, rather than close to together.

Pelvic Bridge with Ball

This version of *Pelvic Bridge* adds a balance challenge.

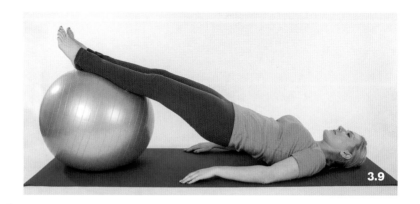

1 Lie on your back on a mat with an exercise ball placed underneath your calves.

2 During an organizing exhale breath, stabilize your core and lift your pelvis off the mat so you are like a plank from your shoulders to your legs, which are resting on the exercise ball (fig. 3.9).

3 Return to the mat as you breathe in.

4 Repeat the exercise 6 to 8 times.

You will quickly notice the added balance challenge of doing this exercise with your legs on a ball. Use your core muscles for balance. Remember, the ball will roll in the direction of more pressure, indicating you are pressing more onto one leg. Try to keep the ball still by equally lifting off both legs. The exercise is easier if the ball is close to your body (thighs or knees on the ball), and more difficult when the ball is farther away from your body (calves or ankles on the ball).

Pelvic Bridge with Ball: Balance

**This version of *Pelvic Bridge* adds an additional balance challenge by taking
away support from your arms.**

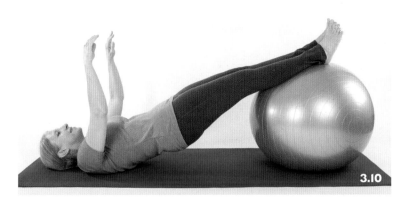

1 Lie on your back on a mat with an exercise ball placed underneath your calves.

2 During an organizing exhale breath, stabilize your core and lift your pelvis off
the mat so you are like a plank from your shoulders to your legs, which are
resting on the exercise ball.

3 Maintain normal breathing as you first bend your elbows so your forearms are
off the mat.

4 If balance is secure, raise your arms completely off the floor (fig. 3.10).

5 Hold this balanced position for several breaths.

6 Return to the mat.

7 Repeat the exercise 3 to 4 times.

Balancing becomes more challenging when you lift your arms. Work to keep
the ball still. Remember, the ball rolls in the direction of increased leg pressure. Use
your core muscles for balance, and your leg muscles for lift.

Pelvic Bridge with Ball: Single Leg

Using a ball and lifting one leg adds another balance challenge to this version of *Pelvic Bridge*.

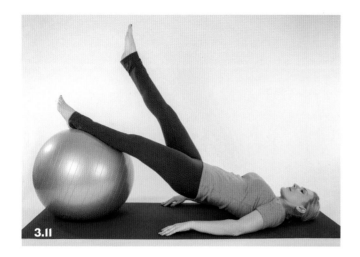

3.11

1 Lie on your back on a mat with an exercise ball placed underneath your calves.

2 During an organizing exhale breath, stabilize your core and lift your pelvis off the mat so you are like a plank from your shoulders to your legs, which are resting on the exercise ball.

3 Carefully shift your left leg toward the center of your body, and either lighten or lift the right leg off the ball (fig. 3.11).

4 Return the right leg to the ball and shift it to the center of your body as you lighten or lift your left leg off the ball.

5 Return your body to the mat.

6 Repeat 3 to 4 times per leg.

Perform this exercise slowly: rushing disrupts balance. Think of "shoring up" the leg that supports you on the ball. Use your core muscles to keep your body balanced.

STRETCHES for Gluteal and Hamstring
Muscles, and External Rotators

It is important to keep flexibility in the strong muscles of the leg, as overly tight
or shortened muscles can contribute to misalignment of the pelvis and interfere
with correct posture. The following stretches work on the *hamstrings, gluteal
muscles,* and *external rotators.*

Hamstring Stretch

**This stretch prevents excess tightness of your hamstring muscle, which
can affect posture.**

1 Lie on your back in neutral spine alignment.

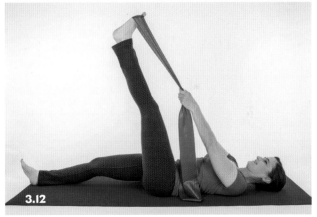

2 Place a towel or stretch band around one foot
and reach that foot to the ceiling, working for
a straight knee (fig. 3.12).

3 Support your leg weight in the stretch band
with your arms, so your leg muscles are not
working to keep your leg in the air. Apply gentle

3.12

traction to your leg—nothing extreme! Do not let your back flatten to the floor.

4 Flex your foot for added calf stretch.

5 Hold for 20 to 30 seconds; repeat with your other leg.

Hamstring Stretch: Standing

I prefer to stretch the hamstrings by lying on the floor, as described on p. 97. Here is an alternate way to do this stretch, however, should you find yourself in a situation where lying down would be difficult.

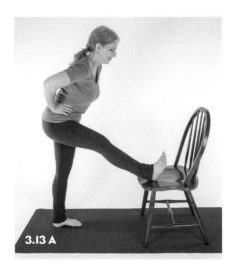 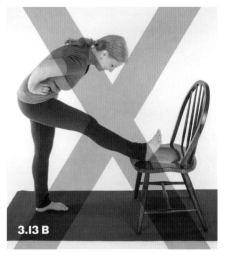

3.13 A   3.13 B

1 Standing upright, rest the heel of your right foot on the edge of a chair or an object of similar height. Straighten your leg.

2 Carefully bend your body forward at the hip joint to accomplish the hamstring stretch (fig. 3.13 A).

3 Hold the stretch for 20 to 30 seconds.

4 Repeat with your left leg.

Do not round your back (fig. 3.13 B), which avoids the hamstring stretch and risks straining your low back. Work to keep neutral spine alignment.

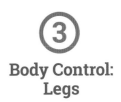
Deep Rotator, Piriformis Stretch

**This stretch combats tightness in the deep rotator
muscles of your hip joint.**

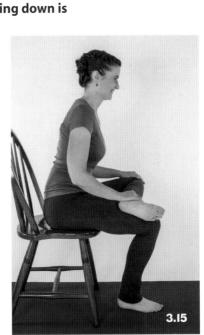

1 Lie on your back, knees bent, feet flat on the floor, in
neutral spine alignment.

2 Place the side of your right foot on the front of your left
thigh, as if crossing your legs.

3 Lift your left leg toward your chest (fig. 3.14). You will
feel the stretch deep in the gluteal region of your right leg.

4 Hold for 20 to 30 seconds.

5 Switch leg positions and repeat.

Deep Rotator, Piriformis Stretch: Sitting

**An alternate way to perform the Deep Rotator Stretch when lying down is
not possible.**

1 Sit upright on a chair. Place your left foot on your right
thigh, as if crossing your legs. Sometimes this position alone
accomplishes a stretch deep in the muscles of your left hip joint.

2 Carefully lean forward from your hip joint (fig. 3.15). This
should deepen the stretch in your left gluteal region. Avoid
rounding your back as you lean forward; this reduces the stretch.

3 Hold the stretch for 20 to 30 seconds.

4 Repeat with the right leg.

A Pretty Picture

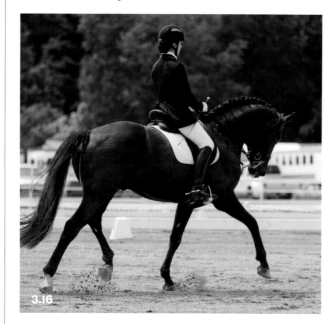

3.16

Catherine Reid shows no evidence of excess leg tension riding Skywalker HW's trot. She sits centered in the saddle, balanced with Skywalker's movement. You get a sense in this photo that she could give away a rein and not lose her balance, also that she can easily use her legs to encourage engagement without causing negative tension in her legs or body. Catherine has found this necessary to keep Skywalker active. He takes offense if her aids become too strong or do not let go. Catherine's body control comes from her ability to separate core stability from hip-joint suppleness, which is taught in the Knee Circles and Leg Circles exercises.

RIDER'S CHALLENGE

Overusing Gluteal Muscles

Linda brings her horse, Wendberg, to the large outdoor arena. The rider's slight build is in distinct contrast to the gelding's stocky frame. During their warm-up, I see Wendberg's blasé attitude force Linda to work and work to keep him going. Linda resorts to using her gluteal muscles to "push" Wendberg into an active walk, with minimal response. Linda pushes harder with her glutes, but Wendberg hardly changes. It is not until Linda gives a thwack with the whip that the gelding becomes lively, at least, for a short time. The same pattern appears in the posting trot, with Linda exaggerating the forward thrust of her pelvis at the top of the rise, trying to keep Wendberg moving. And at canter, Linda pushes each stride with a pronounced forward-back movement of her pelvis.

Linda presents a classic picture of a rider working harder than the horse and using her gluteal muscles in a counterproductive manner. Linda understands her dilemma, "I've had such a problem figuring how *not* to use my butt muscles so much. If not them, what do I use?"

Remedy

I coach Linda to use just her lower leg to get Wendberg going. I suggest a quick, bright leg aid, not a long squeezing one. Wendberg will likely tune out a long squeezing aid, leaving Linda working harder and harder with little to show for her effort. A squeezing aid locks her legs against Wendberg's movement and contributes to his sluggish way of going.

Adductors and Abductors

The *adductors* (grippers) and *abductors* (anti-grippers) are two muscle groups with opposite action. The *adductors* pull the leg *to* the middle of the body, and the *abductors* pull the leg *away* from the middle of the body.

The *adductors* are the inner-thigh muscles. A group of five strong muscles (fig. 3.17), the adductors attach to the pubic bone and along the inside of the thighbone. The action of the adductors pulls the thigh against the saddle; as such, they are often overused to grip the saddle like a clothespin. Certainly, the adductors are important to stabilize proper leg position, but their role must not expand to include security.

The *abductors* work in the opposite way: They pull the thigh away from the saddle. As such, they help stabilize the position of the thighbone (femur).

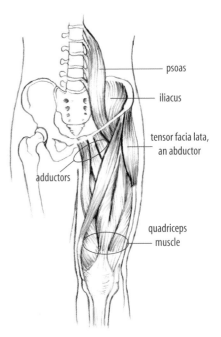

3.17 *The anterior thigh muscles.*

psoas

iliacus

tensor facia lata, an abductor

adductors

quadriceps muscle

I stand by Wendberg's left shoulder facing his rear and place my hands around Linda's left boot heel. I tell her to give my hands a "leg aid" by using her hamstring muscle to pull her lower leg back. I am careful to not have her do this against Wendberg's side, as she would be giving Wendberg a leg aid without expecting a response from him—and that would be bad training indeed!

Linda's initial response is to try and press her lower leg directly into Wendberg's side. This motion causes her leg to externally rotate and her gluteal muscles to fire, and she is pinged out of the saddle. I cue her to think of using the hamstring muscles to pull her leg *back,* not in. And to avoid engaging the gluteal muscles, I have her think of the effort coming farther down on her leg, or closer to the back of the knee. This helps separate the action of the hamstring muscles from the glutes. By imagining her heel being directed toward the

fetlock of Wendberg's opposite hind leg, Linda feels her hamstring muscle engage, and I feel a stronger, clearly defined movement against my hands. She is able to give a clear "on" and "off" aid. We repeat the exercise with her right leg.

Back on the rail, Linda practices applying quick and short lower-leg aids. This allows her to keep her glutes soft and her entire leg swinging with Wendberg's side. Wendberg quickly learns to respect the quicker leg aid, but when he loses activity and slows down, Linda struggles not to use her glutes. As she practices using her leg in this new way, however, Linda gives a clearer leg aid, lightens her workload, and allows Wendberg to respond with a freer gait.

Exercises for Linda: *Pelvic Rocking Supine; Pelvic Rocking on Ball: Front to Back; Pelvic Bridge: Simple, Single leg, and with Ball.*

The following exercises improve awareness, strength, and control of your *adductor* and *abductor* muscles. As well, stretches are described to keep these muscles supple.

Ball Tongs: Squeezes
Works the adductors (grippers).

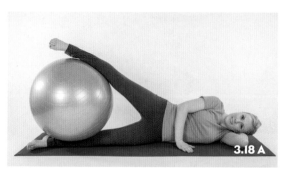

1 Lie on your left side, holding an exercise ball between your lower legs (fig. 3.18 A).

2 Rest your head on your left arm on the mat, and place your right hand on the floor in front of your waist for balance.

3 Check that your body is properly aligned, with your shoulders stacked one upon the other and your pelvis lined up perpendicular to the floor. Straighten your legs and place them at a slight angle in front of the rest of your body.

4 On an exhale breath, squeeze the ball between your legs (fig. 3.18 B), then release the squeeze on the inhale breath.

5 Repeat 6 to 8 times, then switch sides.

Be careful that your spine doesn't twist during the leg movements. Keep your weight centered over the left side of your pelvis. For added difficulty, remove your supporting hand from the mat.

Ball Tongs: Lifts
Works the abductors (anti-grippers).

1 Lie on your left side, holding an exercise ball between your lower legs (fig. 3.19 A).

2 Rest your head on your left arm on the mat, and place your right hand on the floor in front of your waist for balance.

3 Check that your body is properly aligned, with your shoulders stacked one upon the other and your pelvis lined up perpendicular to the floor. Straighten your legs on a line slightly in front of the rest of your body.

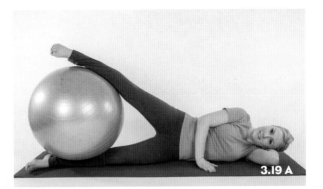

4 On an exhale breath, lift the ball and legs together off the mat; use your right arm for support, if needed (fig. 3.19 B). Rest your legs back down on the inhale breath.

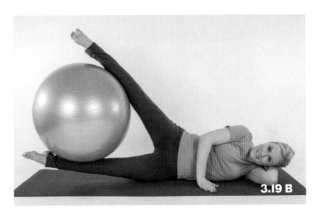

5 Repeat 6 to 8 times, then switch sides.

Be careful that your spine doesn't twist during the leg movements. Keep your weight centered over the left side of your pelvis. For added difficulty, remove your supporting hand from the mat.

Adductor Stretch

Combats tightness in the adductor muscles of the hip joint.

1 Lie on your back on a mat.

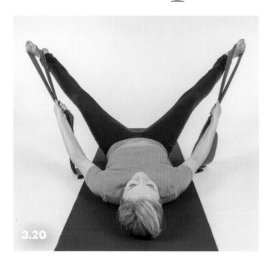

3.20

2 Wrap a towel or elastic stretch band around the bottom of each foot.

3 Hold tightly on to the towels or bands while reaching your legs together up toward the ceiling, as straight as possible, and then carefully supporting them in a stretch out to the side (fig. 3.20). Be sure to avoid changing your pelvic position during this stretch.

4 Hold for 20 to 30 seconds.

RIDER'S CHALLENGE ||||||||||||||||||||||||||||||||||||||||||||||||||||||||||||||||||||||||||||||||||||||||||||||||||||||||||||

Gripping Adductors

Before working with a new rider, I ask her to provide some information about her riding experience, goals, and how I might help her. On her form, Elise states, "I don't understand why I get so tired after only riding about 30 minutes. I do not think I'm that out of shape!"

I meet Elise on her six-year-old bay Trakehner mare, Peony, and watch her do some warm-up rounds at posting trot and canter. She has a reasonably correct posture and rides with a very positive "come with me" attitude. However, while the mare will initially pick up the canter fairly readily, before long Peony loses impulsion and breaks out of canter.

"It is so much work to keep her going!" Elise exclaims as she comes back to a walk.

I have Elise do some trot work first to sort out the challenge she has keeping Peony moving in canter. At posting trot, Elise maintains good balance and alignment and stays with Peony. At sitting trot, however, it is a challenge for Elise to keep Peony in a rhythmic and ground-covering trot. I see that Elise's leg gets quite still—too still—and that her back loses its stable position. Her leg position gets so locked that her feet bounce up and down in the stirrup, rather than rest on the stirrup with movement through the ankle joints.

Elise grips hard to keep from bouncing at sitting trot. By doing so, she inhibits Peony's movement, interfering with her staying in a good trot. I'm suspicious that this is also what is going on in the canter. I explain to Elise that her legs should be against the horse, but not gripping. When the legs grip, it is like riding with the brakes on. Peony responds with a loss of steadiness in the trot and a tendency to break out of the canter.

Abductor Stretch

To combat tightness in the abductor muscles of the outer hip joint. I often
do this stretch right after the Hamstring Stretch (p. 97).

1 Support your right leg in either a stretch band or a
towel, holding it with your left hand.

2 Reach your leg as straight as possible to the ceiling
(like the *Hamstring Stretch*).

3 Let your right leg go left across your left thigh, without
much change in your pelvic position (fig. 3.21).

4 Hold the stretch for 20 to 30 seconds.

5 Repeat with your left leg.

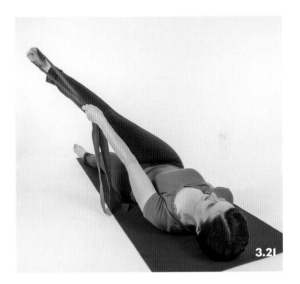

3.21

Remedy

At the halt, I have Elise actively stabilize her spine with her deep abdominal and back muscles, then carefully lift her legs slightly away from the saddle, out to the side. She immediately feels how much heavier she sits in the saddle, in a good way. I have her repeat the exercise at walk to help her learn the sensation of a more supple, less-gripping leg, and a heavier and more anchored position of her pelvis. I emphasize that it is easy to strain her back with this exercise of lifting the legs off the saddle; it must be done carefully with suitable spine support, aiming for a small range of upper-thigh motion, as if she were trying to slide a piece of paper between her leg and the horse.

Back at sitting trot, I again coach Elise to activate her core muscles and then try a few steps of sitting trot, keeping her legs far enough "away" from the saddle to prevent gripping. She does this for a few steps, and then her legs fire. But she begins to feel when the gripping creeps in.

We do the same exercise at canter to try and get her legs to let go and allow Peony to canter freely. To prevent her legs from clinging to Peony's side, I coach her to give a fairly loose leg aid, being conscious of its beginning and end: Apply the aid and then *let go*. I also tell Elise to, at times, give a light tap with the whip, rather than use a leg aid, to encourage Peony to stay in canter. In this way, Elise feels her legs stay released and free.

Our lesson lasts about 45 minutes, with a lot of transitions and attempts to keep Elise's leg muscles supple and not gripping at all gaits. At the end Elise remarks, "I don't remember the last time I rode for 45 minutes straight through without a break."

Exercises for Elise: *Knee Circles; Leg Circles; Leg Lifts on Ball*.

A Pretty Picture

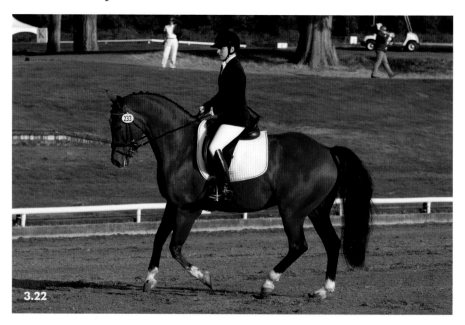

3.22

Jessica Rattner has a released leg position in canter on "V." As previously described (see p. 20), this sensitive horse requires Jessica to ride with tact. Here, he is a bit strong in the canter and Jessica is working to keep a stable position of her pelvis despite his resistance through the left rein. Were Jessica to grip with her legs during this moment, it is likely that V's neck tension would get worse. Jessica patiently guides V to a better connection by staying balanced, supple in her leg muscles, and tactful with her rein aids. To be perfect, I'd encourage Jessica to try and sit a bit more back, with her pelvis secure to the saddle. She notes, however, that V's canter is like a roller coaster! Helpful exercises to develop this stability and tactfulness include any exercises for core strength (such as Abdominal Curls; Crisscross; Quadruped: Single; Quadruped: Diagonal; Plank on Mat: Knees or Plank on Mat: Feet); leg-suppleness exercises (Knee Circles and/or Leg Circles); and arm-suppleness exercises (Hug-a-Tree and Partner Arm Suppleness).

Quadriceps

In Figure 3.17 (p. 101), note the large *quadriceps* muscle that forms the bulk of the front of the thigh. One of the strongest muscles in the body, this muscle has four parts (hence the name). Its primary action is to straighten the knee, but one part of the muscle crosses the hip joint and can flex this joint (along with the *iliopsoas* muscles). The quadriceps muscle can interfere with hip-joint mobility by pulling the knee up against the knee roll of the saddle. And the quadriceps muscle can disrupt leg position (see "The Rider's Challenge: Unstable Leg Position in Posting," p. 171). The quadriceps muscle does not do much while you are riding. It is not common to straighten the knee joint in the saddle. Two exceptions are the "up" phase of posting trot and correcting the position of a lower leg that is too far back.

EXERCISE for Quadriceps Muscle

Straight Legs
Strengthen the quadriceps muscle.

1 Lie on your back, holding an exercise ball between your feet.

2 Bend your hip joint so that your femur (thighbone) is perpendicular to the floor, and bend your knee joint so that your lower leg is parallel to the floor. Keep your spine in neutral alignment. Place your arms by your sides or use your hands to support your thighbone position (fig. 3.23 A).

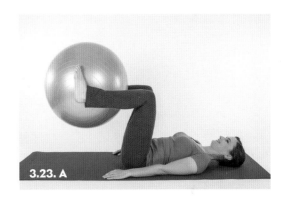

3.23. A

3 Take an inhale breath, and on the exhale straighten your legs at the knee joint; keep your hip joint stable (fig. 3.23 B).

4 Return to start position on an inhale breath.

5 Repeat 6 to 8 times.

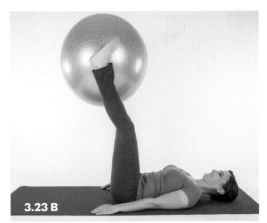

3.23 B

If your hamstrings are tight, you may not be able to completely straighten your knee joint. This is okay. Do not compensate for this by letting your thighs fall away from your body. Be sure to keep your femur perpendicular to the floor so you do not strain your back. Your spine alignment should not change during the exercise.

Hamstring Support Reduces Knee Pain

Roberta is an enthusiastic adult amateur rider who enjoys both dressage and eventing. She started riding after having children, and the sport joined her list of other activities: running, hiking, downhill skiing, bike riding. Her active life, however, is taking its toll on her body, and she recently underwent arthroscopic knee surgery on her left knee for a torn meniscus. After post-operative recovery and physical therapy, she and I work together in the studio to help her regain core strength and develop improved leg alignment and body balance.

When she is able to return to riding, she experiences knee pain when she rides posting trot and two-point position in her jumping saddle. She is concerned she'll have to give up jumping and does not want to do that. She comes for a riding session to see if we can sort out what is causing her pain.

Roberta arrives for her lesson in her jump saddle. While she warms up she keeps me apprised of when her knee hurts. Consistently, she notes knee pain when her left foot slips too far forward. This happens when her horse startles or hurries, and sometimes when she gives an aid with her left leg.

I have two ideas that could be causing a problem for Roberta. First, like many riders, she tries to pull her calf directly into the horse's side to give a leg aid. Since the knee does not move this way, she is forced to externally rotate her thighbone at her hip joint, causing rotational strain across her knee. Second, the quadriceps muscle on the front of the thigh is the muscle primarily engaged when Roberta straightens her knee and pushes her foot forward. I am suspicious that her knee pain comes from the subsequent pressure exerted on the patella (knee cap) along with the necessary inward gripping from her adductors associated with this unstable leg position.

Remedy

First, we review how to give a leg aid. I encourage focusing on the hamstrings to press her calf back to her horse's opposite hind-leg fetlock.

I also have Roberta post out of the saddle several times at halt, guiding her to stabilize her foot position with her hamstring muscle in the back of her thigh. This prevents her foot from sliding forward and keeps a suitable bend in her knee. I have her think that when she posts the trot, her horse lifts her through the back of her thigh, bringing her pelvis forward over the pommel of the saddle. This helps her focus on the hamstrings, and keeps her feet underneath her. To demonstrate how unstable she is when her foot comes forward, I move her left foot (the leg of her operated knee) slightly forward. Roberta falls back in the saddle (as I suspect she will) and exclaims "Ouch!" I apologize profusely for causing her pain, but we both agree that her response clarifies that her forward-foot position is part of the issue.

We spend the rest of the lesson practicing posting trot and two-point position making sure that her feet stay underneath her body. She focuses on engaging her hamstring muscles for improved leg stability. (In fact, she later tells me they were a bit sore the next day.) Off-horse exercises for Roberta: the *Pelvic Bridge* exercise series.

Iliopsoas Muscle

Figure 3.24 shows the *iliopsoas* (pronounced il-e-o-'so-az) muscle. It is a unique muscle in that it is the only muscle that connects the femur directly to the vertebrae (spine) at the center of the body. All other thigh muscles connect the femur to the pelvis. Its muscle fibers insert on either side of the low thoracic and upper-lumbar spine where the muscle is called just the *psoas*. From there it courses through the pelvis, being joined by the *iliacus* muscle, and is called the *iliopsoas*. It then inserts on the top of the femur.

The iliopsoas muscle is a strong hip flexor. That is, it lifts your knee toward your chest, decreasing the angle of your hip joint in the front of your body. Since it attaches to the spine, the iliopsoas can also extend (arch) the spine.

The iliopsoas lies deep within the body: It is not easily felt and cannot be seen. As such, it is a hard muscle to understand. Those who have tight and restricting psoas muscles have perhaps had massage or physical therapy to loosen the muscle and know the intense feeling of the muscle being massaged through the abdominal wall.

As a strong and central muscle, the iliopsoas can work for you or against you. When supple and controlled, the iliopsoas muscle offers both spine and hip-joint stability with refined control of motion and leg position. This positive function requires control of spine alignment with the postural muscles (which I discussed in chapter 2).

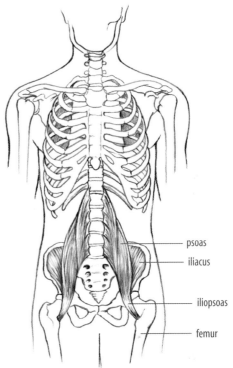

psoas
iliacus

iliopsoas

femur

3.24 *The iliopsoas muscle. Note that it originates as the psoas on either side of the spine, enters the pelvis where it is joined by the iliacus muscle of the pelvis to become the iliopsoas muscle, and then attaches to the top of the femur.*

EXERCISES for Iliopsoas Muscle

The following *Knee Folds* exercise integrates spine stability with iliopsoas muscle function.

Knee Folds

Coordinate the function of the iliopsoas muscle with your core muscles.

1 Lie on the floor, knees bent, feet flat on the floor hip-joint width apart.

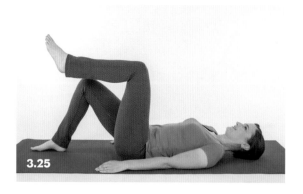

2 Take an inhale breath, and then exhale and pull in your lower abdominal muscles to stabilize your spine.

3 Lift your left knee toward your chest (fig. 3.25), and set your leg back down without letting your pelvis rock side to side.

4 Repeat with your right leg, doing 6 to 8 leg lifts per side.

3.25

RIDER'S CHALLENGE ||||||||||||||||||||||||||||||||||||||||||||||||||||||||||||||||||||||||||||||||||||||||||||||||||||

Tight Iliopsoas Muscle

Sarah jogs up on Trapper as I arrive at her outdoor arena. "I have an important issue to discuss today," she says. "It is embarrassing, but lately after I ride I am sore where I sit in the saddle, and oh my, it hurts to pee after riding!"

Sarah is an advanced beginning amateur rider who recently started leasing this 12-year-old Hanoverian schoolmaster. She is having some difficulty adjusting to his large gaits and learning to stay with his movement.

I watch Sarah at walk and posting trot. Her focus and postural alignment and balance are quite satisfactory. When she tries to sit Trapper's large trot, however, I see her knees pull up and in against the knee roll of the saddle, and her torso comes forward with an arch in her spine. She bounces madly, making the gripping worse. Trapper stiffens his back and loses impulsion.

I explain a little bit about the iliopsoas muscle. I believe this muscle is pulling her thighbone up causing too much flexion at her hip joint, and pulling her lumbar spine forward in extension (arching) in an attempt to stabilize her balance. It is not an uncommon strategy, but unfortunately, it doesn't work well: It pulls her pelvic floor uncomfortably onto the front of the saddle, causes fatigue, and interferes with Trapper's way of going.

Engage your trunk muscles to prevent your pelvis from rocking and your weight from shifting while you lift each leg. Pay careful attention to your pelvic position during the exercise, and work for complete pelvic stability with no wiggles.

To access the ilipsoas muscle to lift your leg, imagine that the movement comes from deep within your body's center. Because this muscle is deep within your body and you can't really feel it, you only know you are using it correctly if other muscles work less.

You can tell when you access the ilipsoas if the tendon of a more superficial muscle (the *rectus femoris*) at the front of your hip joint barely tightens during this movement. Check for this by placing your thumbs over the front of your hip joint. When this tendon barely pops up, you are accessing the ilipsoas muscle to move your leg. Also, using the ilipsoas muscle for this exercise confers a stable feeling to your body; it becomes easier to prevent the pelvis from rocking side to side during the leg lift, and your leg feels like it weighs less.

This exercise is made more challenging by lifting one knee, and then alternating leg positions, so you always have one leg resting on the mat and one leg in the air.

Remedy

I guide Sarah into a more balanced position with her abdominal muscles supporting neutral spine and pelvic alignment. Like a seat belt, these muscles support the pelvis as if it were laced to the back of the saddle. These same muscles keep the pelvis and pubic bone more supported in the front of Sarah's body, preventing the front of her pelvic floor from pressing uncomfortably on the twist of the saddle. As well, I have her seek a hip angle that is more open or extended, with her knee staying down in the saddle. With her abdominals pressing back toward her spine and her knees reaching down, she is lengthening the iliopsoas muscle and telling the abdominal muscles to take over the work of balance and support that the overworking iliopsoas has provided.

Sarah goes back to the rail to try out these changes. She is able to keep her pelvis anchored with her "seat-belt" abdominals for a few steps, but then she finds herself pitched forward and gripping. It can take some doing to change a habit. I encourage her to try to keep her improved posture for a few steps of a slow sitting trot, and then come to walk when she feels herself start to grip again. With practice, she will eventually sit more and more steps, and then a bigger and bigger trot. Exercises for Sarah: *Pelvic Rocking Supine; Pelvic Rocking on Ball: Front to Back; Knee Folds; and Hip Flexor Stretch.*

Hip Flexor Stretch

Combat tightness in the muscles that flex your hip joint.

1 Kneel on a mat and place your right foot in front of you. You will be resting on your left knee and your right foot. You can use an exercise ball to balance and support your upper body.

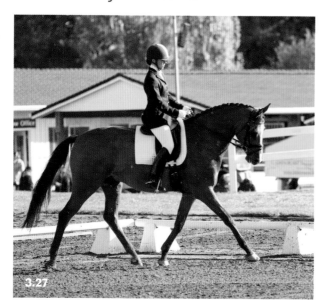

2 Press your weight forward over your right foot (position your right foot so you avoid bending your knee more than 90 degrees). You will feel a stretch in the front of your left thigh (fig. 3.26).

3 Hold the stretch for 20 to 30 seconds; repeat on the right side.

Keep neutral spine alignment and avoid arching your back in the stretch.

3.26

A Pretty Picture

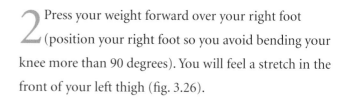

Catherine Reid's long leg and "knee-down" position on Karibbean is evidence of her not gripping up—or in—with her leg muscles. This is something she is constantly aware of. How can you achieve this beautiful long leg on your horse? Learn to separate core stability from leg-muscle tension. It is often very challenging for a rider to feel strong and engaged in the core muscles without leg tension. The work of the core muscles can "generalize" to the leg, causing negative tension in the muscles of the hip joint and a tight, immoveable leg. In all your core exercises, be sure to keep your leg muscles "out of it." Use Knee Circles and Leg Circles to perfect the feeling of core stability with suppleness of the leg.

3.27

Common Leg Position and Function Challenges

In all of us, the weight of the leg comprises a significant portion of our body weight. As such, the legs can have significant unwanted effects on body position and function. Using the leg to aid the horse can alter posture, and overzealous leg muscles can inhibit the horse's motion. Finally, leg position can influence your ability to balance efficiently. These are reasons to keep the legs under control and balanced in strength and flexibility.

Leg Dysfunction Affects Posture

Legs can affect posture in several ways. When you apply a leg aid you can cause your pelvis to tuck under your body, bringing your spine into flexed (rounded or C-shaped) posture. This is especially true if you tend to overuse your gluteal muscles. This can strain your back because force is being applied to your rounded spine. Body awareness and core stability will improve your ability to give a leg aid without such a change in posture. This is one of the components of being able to give *independent aids*. So, work to become aware that leg movement at your hip joint need not change your spine alignment. Off-horse practice like the exercises below will help you differentiate movement of your leg at the hip joint from movement of your pelvis and spine. The *Knee* and *Leg Circles* exercises that follow will help you develop this awareness and skill of core stability with supple movement at the hip joint.

MY CHALLENGE ||||||||||||||||||||||||||||||||||||||||||||||||||

Separate Leg Movement from Spine Movement

It was a huge revelation when, during my Pilates training, I discovered how I had been muddying the movement of my hip joints with the movement of my spine. I had been linking them in a single glob: When I moved or used my legs to walk, lift, or give an aid to my horse, I had no idea that, at the same time, I was flexing (rounding) my lumbar spine. I can't say that this caused my back troubles, but I am sure this habitual movement didn't help. It took time for me to learn to differentiate hip-joint movement from movement at my lumbar spine. The clear teaching of several patient instructors helped me sort this out. With this awareness I became better at keeping my spine stable while letting my legs do their job.

Knee Circles

Learn to separate movement at the hip joint from movement at the spine, and improve spine stability and hip-joint muscle suppleness.

1 Lie on the floor, knees bent, feet flat on the floor hip-joint width apart.

2 On an exhale breath and while keeping neutral spine, lift your right knee toward your chest (fig. 3.28 A). Place your hand on top of your right knee (not shown). Straighten your left leg so it is flat on the mat.

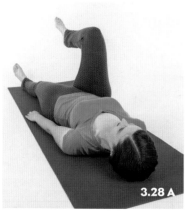

3.28 A

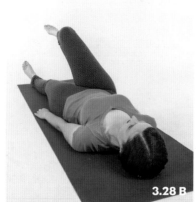

3.28 B

3 On another exhale breath, move your right knee in a circle to the left, bringing the right knee over your left thigh, away from you, out to the right, then inhale as you return your knee to the start position (figs. 3.28 B–D).

4 Do 6 circles left, then 6 circles right.

5 Repeat with your left knee.

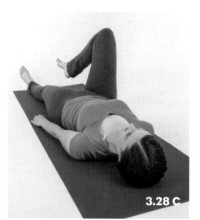

3.28 C

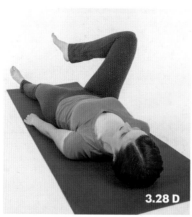

3.28 D

Use your trunk muscles to keep the pelvis stable, unaffected by your leg movement. Do not allow your pelvis or torso to rock side to side as your leg moves. Gradually let go of your knee and do the circles without the help of your hand (as shown in the photo series).

Leg Circles
A further challenge to differentiate movement at the hip joint from movement at the spine. *Leg Circles,* harder to do than *Knee Circles,* also improve spine stability and hip-joint muscle suppleness.

1 Lie on the floor, knees bent, feet flat on the floor hip-joint width apart.

2 On an exhale breath and while keeping neutral spine, lift your right knee toward your chest. Straighten your right leg as much as possible while keeping neutral spine alignment. Straighten your left leg flat on the mat (fig. 3.29 A).

3 On the next exhale breath, move the right leg in a circle left, going across the left thigh, down toward the floor, and slightly out to the right side. Inhale as you return your leg to the start position (fig. 3.29 B–D).

4 Do 6 circles left, then 6 circles right.

5 Repeat with your left leg.

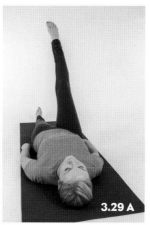
3.29 A

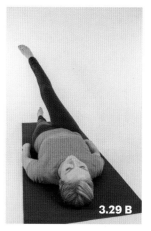
3.29 B

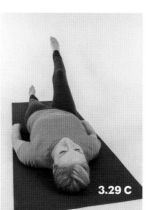
3.29 C

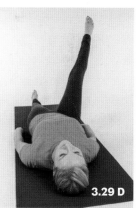
3.29 D

Use your trunk muscles to keep your pelvis stable, unaffected by your leg movement. Do not allow your pelvis or torso to rock side to side as your leg moves. Place your hands on the sides of your pelvis to feel if your pelvis is rocking during the circles. You'll find it particularly challenging to maintain pelvic stability as your leg stretches out to the side.

The *Knee* and *Leg Circle* exercises allow you to feel what it is like to have a stable torso and a mobile hip joint with suppleness in these strong leg muscles. Adjust your circle size (smaller is easier), and keep your pelvis stable while you move your leg. Focus on feeling the stability of your pelvis with coordinated movement of your leg, as you should when riding.

Leg Aids Disrupt Posture

Remember Julie and Bismark from chapter 2, the gelding that needs motivation to move freely (see p. 57)? The first story focuses on Julie's spine alignment, bringing her into a more upright posture with less flexion (rounding) of her spine. This helps her stay balanced with Bismark's large and lanky trot and prevents her from falling behind his movement. The second issue that challenges Julie's posture is the way she applies leg aids. With each leg aid, her rounded posture returns, complicating her balance.

Julie tends to give a "go" aid to Bismark by squeezing her lower leg against his side, and at the same time, squeezing her gluteal muscles. Her gluteal muscles pull her pelvis into a tucked position, rounding her back and pointing her seat bones forward. At halt, I remind Julie of correct posture, then I show her how to apply her lower-leg aid just from the hamstring muscle, without the effort generalizing up into her gluteal muscles. In this way, she avoids rounding her spine into a potentially harmful position.

"But I always hear 'drive him more from your seat,'" she says. "So what should I be doing?"

Remedy

I explain that pumping with the gluteal muscles is not the best way to get a sluggish horse moving. I coach Julie to give quick lower-leg aids, keeping her gluteal muscles less involved, and to have a clear start and finish to each leg aid so her legs can release. This decreases her work and the likelihood that her posture will be disrupted.

Back on the rail, Julie practices her new, quick lower-leg aids. Bismark does not always respond, and Julie then reverts to involving her gluteal muscles and rounding her back. I urge her to use her whip, as opposed to her gluteal muscles, to get Bismark going. Not only will there be clearer consequences to him, but also she'll avoid straining her back by pulling it forcefully out of good alignment.

Exercises for Julie: *Pelvic Rocking Supine; Knee Folds; Knee Circles; Leg Circles; and Leg Lifts on Ball.*

Iliopsoas Dysfunction and Posture

A tight and restricting iliopsoas muscle can also disrupt position. A short iliopsoas muscle will tend to pull the lumbar spine forward and into an arch (extension), and pull the hip joint into flexion, narrowing the hip angle (see the example in The Rider's Challenge: "Tight Iliopsoas Muscle" in this chapter, p. 110). The rider tends to be pitched forward with seat bones pointing too far back. The iliopsoas is a strong muscle, and this forced position of the arched spine (in extension) can cause back strain or worsen facet-joint arthritis. The antidote for this position problem is finding correct neutral spine alignment, supporting this position with the deep abdominal muscles, and allowing the iliopsoas to stretch and lengthen—to take the work of balance away from the iliopsoas muscle. Then, the knee can move downward, increasing the hip joint angle. The image of kneeling can help you get this feeling in the saddle. The *Hip Flexor Stretch* exercise in this chapter can teach you this movement off the horse (p. 112).

A Pretty Picture

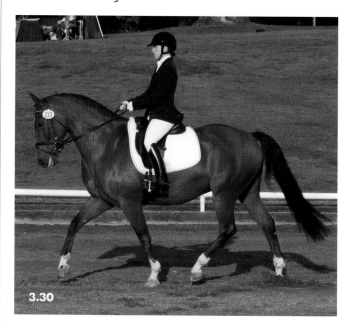

3.30

Jessica Rattner rides "V" freely forward on the centerline. Her lack of leg-muscle tension and correct balance facilitates his gait. V can be quick to predict upcoming movements, so Jessica must have clear "on" and "off" leg aids to keep him from becoming anxious and anticipating the next move. And, any tendency to give leg aids with her gluteal muscles causes V to tighten his back. Jessica finds Pelvic Bridge exercises useful for keeping her leg aids organized. With these exercises, she gains awareness of when her hamstrings engage and when they release, so she can do the same in the saddle as she applies her leg aids.

If your balance is unsteady, moving your leg to apply an aid can disrupt your position and make it difficult for your horse to understand your cue. Torso-muscle support prevents this problem. Pay attention to your torso stability while applying leg aids. This may be particularly important when using a strong leg aid. Think of using the opposite side of your torso to counterbalance the leg aid. The *Leg Lifts on Ball* exercise below will help you develop this skill.

EXERCISE to Learn Core Stability with Leg Movement

Leg Lifts on Ball

Develop the skill of staying balanced while sitting upright and moving one leg; this will help you stay stable in the saddle while giving leg aids.

1 Sit on an exercise ball or a chair in neutral spine alignment, feet flat on the floor hip-joint width apart.

2 Take an easy inhale breath.

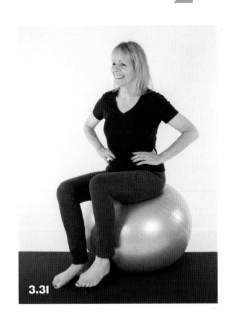

3.31

3 On the exhale breath, support your torso and lift your left leg off the floor, with your knee bent (fig. 3.31), then set it back down as you inhale.

4 Repeat with your right leg. Lift each leg 5 times.

Work to keep your body and pelvis stable on the ball or chair as you lift one leg. It requires tremendous torso stability to remain still while you lift one leg. Feel the cross-body balance that happens: As you lift your left leg, feel the muscles of your right torso activate to stabilize the body, and vice versa with your right leg.

It is quite normal for your body's coordination to be very different on one side versus the other. Often, lifting the leg opposite your strong side is easier (if you are stronger on your right side, it will likely be easier to stabilize balance when lifting your left leg). If you find it hard to lift one leg without sliding off the ball, think of lifting the opposite pelvis a bit, as you do in the *Pelvic Rocking: Side to Side* exercise, before lifting the challenging leg. This will activate the opposite torso for stability.

Leg Dysfunction Is Inefficient

The gluteals are thigh muscles commonly overused in riding. You can see when a rider is overusing her "glutes": She is the one working hard to get her horse to move. Overusing your glutes causes a pumping motion: You tuck your pelvis under as you try to keep the horse going. This problem is most obvious in walk and canter but is also evident in both sitting and posting trots. This pumping is an ineffective method of giving the horse a "go" aid and is sometimes adopted when you are told to "drive with the seat."

As I've talked about before, using your gluteal muscles to encourage your horse is best reserved for a well-trained and sensitive horse that will respond to a small pelvic tuck. Otherwise you end up working harder and harder, using more and more muscle tone, with little response from your horse and not much to show for your effort. The strong gluteal muscle can cause back strain when used this way. And, I've seen sensitive horses lock their back against their rider's tight gluteal muscles with resulting topline tension and loss of purity of rhythm, particularly in the walk. Using your glutes too much "pings" you out of the saddle and prevents you from feeling your horse's body move underneath you.

It is overly simple to say that you shouldn't use your glutes while in the saddle. That is not the case. These muscles assist in leg extension at the hip joint, thus pulling your leg against your horse's side. The point is to avoid using *only* your glutes to get a sluggish horse going. You'll work too hard with little effect. Instead, use a "go" aid from your lower leg and back it up with a tap of your whip; clearly release the aid so your muscles let go, your hip joint unlocks, you preserve good posture, and your horse can move.

Constantly nagging your horse with leg aids is also inefficient. A lazy horse can coax you into giving a "go" aid with your lower leg every stride. This is a problem of training, one that takes a great deal of rider discipline to correct. Work to have a system of increasing leg aids. Each time you give an aid, start with the little aid, and then increase the forcefulness of the aid until you get a response, perhaps resorting to a tap with a whip. Then, stop giving the aid and expect your horse to continue in the manner that you want.

If your horse loses energy, repeat this routine. Breaking the habit of nagging aids requires you to focus on what you want and be consistent in your system of aids. Every leg aid should have a beginning and an end: a purpose and an outcome.

RIDER'S CHALLENGE |||||||||||||||||||||||||||||||||||||||||||||||||||||||||||||||||||||||||||||||||||||||||||||||||

Avoiding Sacroiliac Strain

Lisa rides a 10-year-old Belgian/Thoroughbred cross gelding, Kaspar. She loves Kaspar's mellow personality, but struggles sometimes to keep him active, especially in canter. Further, she has recently experienced buttock pain during her rides. Her physician believes her pain is from dysfunction of her sacroiliac joint. She contacts me to see if I can identify position or function problems that might contribute to her pain.

Lisa is warming up Kaspar at working trot rising when I arrive at her arena. She stops next to me and while rubbing her left gluteal area says, "I am glad you are here today, already I'm getting some soreness in my left hip region."

I watch Lisa warm up for a few more minutes. I see several factors that could contribute to her SI pain. First, as you might expect from his breeding, Kaspar has a very broad barrel. To ride him, Lisa's legs need to have more external rotation than if she were riding

a more narrow horse. Lisa also adopts a strategy of encouraging Kaspar to move forward by squeezing her gluteal muscles every trot stride (much like Linda on Wendberg in The Rider's Challenge: "Overusing Gluteal Muscles," p. 100). Added to this, Lisa tends to sit heavily on her left seat bone, with her right pelvis lifted up and pulled forward.

At halt, I have Lisa show me how she applies a leg aid. Like many riders, she tries to pull her lower leg directly against Kaspar's side. Added to this, her gluteal muscles engage. Both of these strategies increase the external rotation of her thigh bone; another potential SI strain.

Remedy

"Apply your leg aid with more of the back of your calf," I coach, "so you use the hamstring muscles on the back of your leg. You'll get much more power from your leg aid, and less potential stress across your SI joint. Be careful to not overuse your gluteal muscles to drive Kaspar forward—focus on using your lower leg."

Sometimes it is difficult to be aware that you are, in fact, giving a leg aid every stride or two to keep your horse going. If you think this is the case, try this exercise for a few strides: Pull your legs very slightly away from your horse's sides (to be sure you are not giving aids), and only use a tap with a whip to keep your horse going. This exercise will improve awareness of your leg function, but I do not suggest riding like this all the time, of course. It allows you to feel what it is like for your legs to be supple and released, moving with your horse, and not constantly giving an aid. Try to return to this "released" feeling each time you use your legs to aid your horse.

How often do you hear "Don't grip"? Why is gripping a bad thing? Your leg muscles are strong and can be quite effective, in the short term, at keeping

---

Before Lisa returns to riding, I help her adjust her lateral balance in the saddle. By lifting up the left side of her pelvis, she feels the relief of tension on her right side, and feels her weight settle onto her right seat bone. This change in her pelvic position improves its balance, both right to left and front to back—changes that could decrease SI strain. At sitting trot, Lisa and I work on establishing a more securely balanced pelvic position, left to right. I remind her to give leg aids that come more from her hamstrings and less from her gluteal muscles so as to not disrupt pelvic position. Lisa appreciates that Kaspar moves more freely forward, and she feels less tension in the muscles of her hip joint.

We then tackle her more challenging gait: canter. The right lead is most difficult for her, and I can see why. Her lateral-balance issue becomes more prominent, with her weight shifting to the left (the outside). Her pelvis twists so that the right side comes forward, with upward tension from her hip flexors in her right leg. Her left leg aids make her leftward sitting worse because her left leg falls quite far back, muscling Kaspar forward.

"This definitely gives me pain on my left hip!" Lisa exclaims as she comes back to trot and then walk. We review lateral balance of the pelvis and a more balanced leg position with less extreme use of her gluteal muscles on her left leg.

"Keep your left side short, shifting your weight onto your right seat bone. That will help balance your pelvic and leg positions. Then, apply your left leg aid less far back, with less gluteal muscles," I coach. She tries these strategies, and finds her hip pain does not increase, as it ordinarily would during a ride.

Lisa has several potential contributing factors to her SI pain while riding: her horse's conformation, her lateral imbalance, and the imbalanced function of her right leg (hip flexor dominant) and left leg (gluteal dominant). It is not simple to change out the horse Lisa rides, but paying attention to core and leg function will hopefully decrease her SI strain (see more about this on p. 127).

Exercises for Lisa: *Pelvic Rocking: Side to Side; Pelvic Bridge; Hamstring Stretch; Leg Lifts on Ball; Hip Flexor Stretch.*

you in the saddle: If your horse bucks or bolts, gripping can prevent a fall. But, otherwise, gripping restricts movement at your hip joint and locks your body against the movement of your horse. This has two undesired consequences: It results in unhealthy mechanics in your body and inhibits your horse's movement.

If you grip, you lock or limit motion at your hip joint, and it cannot move with your horse. Your horse's movement must be transferred into your body someplace, and the likely place is the joints of your spine and/or sacroiliac (SI) joint. Gripping can cause excessive and unhealthy movement of these joints.

Recall the description of the cushioning discs that lie between each vertebrae of your spine. These discs allow for some movement between the vertebrae, but if your back moves too much, you risk wear and tear on these discs as well as the facet and SI joints. This is particularly noticeable in the sitting trot. These joints can suffer strain and inflammation from the concussion of your body weight if you bounce against the saddle with a locked hip joint. Most assuredly, there is some movement at these joints while riding all gaits, but if all motion from your horse is absorbed at these joints, you risk strain. By achieving balance and stability in your torso, you support these joints and allow motion to occur at your hip and other leg joints—joints that are meant to move!

Gripping with your legs for balance works against riding efficiently. While riding, the primary function of your legs is to move with, and aid, your horse. Your legs should feel part of your horse's body (see fig. 3.1). A tight leg makes it difficult to feel your horse's movement, and if your leg muscles are busy keeping you secure in the saddle, they are not available for small or subtle leg aids. Your horse will experience a lot of "noise" coming from your gripping legs and will be hard pressed to "hear" your leg aids. You, therefore, will need to give an overly strong aid that your horse can perceive over the white noise of your gripping legs. Further, your horse's natural movement involves his body and rib cage. If your legs grip against this movement, you are telling your horse to stop. Essentially, you are riding with the brakes on, and again, this will require you to give leg aids that are perhaps stronger than necessary.

A Pretty Picture

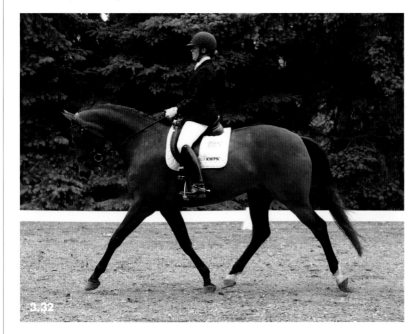

3.32

Lisa Boyer shows a balanced leg position on Zamora. Zamora is a "less is more" horse—that is, if Lisa is careful when applying her leg aids and avoids tension, Zamora's movement improves. You can gain this leg-muscle control with off-horse exercises that develop your awareness of leg-muscle function, such as Pelvic Bridge, Leg Circles, and Knee Folds.

A sure sign of too much leg tone and gripping is fatigue (as in Elise's case—see The Rider's Challenge: "Gripping Adductors" p. 104). The large leg muscles use a lot of energy. Your leg muscles tire when you use them for both balance and loud, strong leg aids. Transferring the work of balance back to your torso allows you to maintain a secure position, ride with less fatigue, and not work your legs so hard.

Besides causing fatigue, overactive leg muscles impair your ability to sit deeply in the saddle. Have you ever been coached to "sit deep" and wondered how to do this? You cannot push yourself into the saddle, you can only sit as heavily or deeply in the saddle as your body weight allows. However, you have many ways to pop yourself out of the saddle. Tight gluteal muscles push you out of the saddle, and gripping adductor muscles ping you out of the saddle. So when you are told to "sit deep," remind your core muscles to secure balance and take work away from your tight leg muscles. Then, let those muscles release—welcome to your saddle!

Leg Aids Disrupt Balance

"I'm having trouble getting Bentley into the canter," Mary explains at our lesson. "He just runs off in the trot, and I can't stay with him."

Mary is thrilled to have a horse with some training. A seven-year-old Warmblood, Bentley is well started and trained to Second Level. Mary, an intermediate rider, is relearning timing and balance in the saddle after taking a break from riding to start a family. What she lacks in body control she makes up for in focus and determination.

Mary and Bentley move off in posting trot. Bentley gets a bit strong and quick in the trot, and Mary responds by pressing into her feet and "water skiing" against the bridle to slow him down. Her body, as a result, is behind his motion, encouraging him onto his forehand.

I coach Mary to breathe and center, and feel more control and balance coming from her torso. By getting her feet underneath her body, her balance improves. I have her ride some 15-meter circles to help steady Bentley and create a trot where he stays underneath her. Mary sits Bentley's trot for a few strides and then asks for the canter. As she had predicted, Bentley runs into a faster trot. Mary's aids are unclear. She thrusts her inside leg forward and turns it out almost as if she were giving an aid to his shoulder. This pushes her pelvis to the back of the saddle; she compensates by leaning forward. Mary's outside leg moves quite far back, contributing to her balance challenge. Bentley, off balance, wonders what to do.

Remedy

I coach Mary to keep her legs more underneath her body when asking for the canter by applying her inside leg by the girth, not in front of it, and her outside leg just behind the girth. I also advise her to not lean forward. She should expect Bentley to canter underneath her.

Mary returns to the rail and tries to modify her leg and body position in the canter transition. While Bentley is still a bit reluctant, Mary's balance is less disrupted and she can more easily correct his running trot. After a few tries, Bentley offers a more prompt canter depart.

Exercises for Mary: *Quadruped: Single; Knee Circles; Leg Circles; Leg Lifts on Ball.*

A Pretty Picture

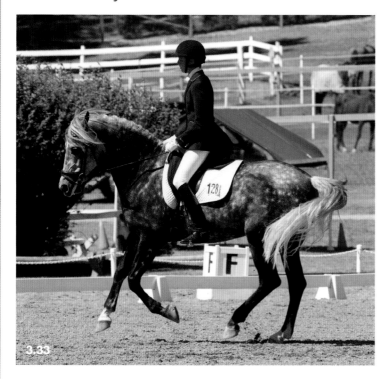

3.33

Garyn Heidemann rides Gabriel in left canter with a correct leg position underneath the center of her body. This good posture allows Garyn to give light, controlled, encouraging leg aids to keep Gabriel's canter jumping. Garyn describes Gabriel as "light and sensitive." He takes offense at random leg aids, but rewards Garyn with a steady, balanced canter when she is steady and balanced in her position. "Otherwise," she says, "he'll get tight in his neck and back and maybe throw in a flying change!" Exercises that are helpful for Garyn include Plank on Mat: Knees or Plank on Mat: Feet (for core stability), and Knee Circles or Leg Circles (for leg control).

About Your Body: **Bursitis**

Several joints in the body have synovial fluid-filled sacs, or *bursae*, that cushion and allow movement of tendons over bone. When healthy, the bursae promote fluid, pain-free movement. These bursae are located in the knee, hip, shoulder, elbow, heel, and around the seat bones *(ischial tuberosities)* of the pelvis.

Bursitis is inflammation of these bursae. It can result from trauma, or from excessive pressure on a bursa from overuse and/or unbalanced muscle function. The end result of the inflammation is pain and stiffness in the affected joint. Treatments are geared at reducing the inflammation, and then preventing aggravation with movement education. Riders who have bursitis must be careful to use the muscles of the affected joint in balance to limit excess pressure.

Leg Muscle Imbalance Aggravates Bursitis

Heather owns a 14-year-old Thoroughbred gelding named Jester, and divides her riding time between dressage, work over fences, and trail riding. I have worked with Heather several times, mostly on body control. Today she arrives with a specific concern.

"I've been seeing a physical therapist for pain in my left hip joint. My doctor thinks it is bursitis. Riding, especially jumping, is making it worse. I'm hoping you can help me sort out what I'm doing that irritates my hip joint," she says.

I observe Heather at walk and posting trot. She notes that her hip is a bit irritated. The first issue I see is that Heather overuses her gluteal muscles when asking her horse to go more forward. At the walk, she is clenching these muscles every step. In addition, each time she gives a leg aid, her knee is pulled away from the saddle flap. I am concerned that the external (outward) rotation of her thighbone at the hip joint with the force of these leg aids is triggering the irritation of the joint.

At the halt, I have Heather demonstrate how she gives a leg aid against my hand. She tries to apply her calf directly inward. Since the knee is a hinge joint and cannot accomplish this movement, her thigh externally rotates at the hip joint. This fires her gluteal muscles. Not good.

Remedy

As an alternative method of giving a leg aid, I have Heather pull her heel back and toward the fetlock on her horse's opposite hind leg. This allows her knee to bend (flex) slightly, and utilizes more of the hamstring muscle for the leg aid with less use of her gluteal muscles and less external rotation at her hip joint. She is amazed at the improved control she has of her leg using this technique. I also encourage Heather to avoid constantly giving leg aids: Each leg aid should have a clear beginning and a clear end. This will improve her horse's responsiveness and help her avoid chronic leg-muscle tension that could contribute to her hip pain.

It is extremely challenging for Heather not to use her gluteal muscles to "push" Jester forward every step at the walk. I have Heather squeeze her gluteal muscles firmly and then let them release. She feels how deeply she can sit in the saddle after the muscles release. I encourage her to keep that feeling of her weight being grounded in the saddle as her baseline position. This exercise improves her awareness of when the gluteal muscles are overactive.

Heather remarks that the reduced gluteal-muscle tension at the walk makes her hip joint less irritated. Heather moves on to sitting trot, where again she tries to "create" every step with her gluteal muscles and becomes very tight in her legs. We keep the trot slow and manageable to help Heather keep her legs released. This is always my strategy when working to change riding habits. Make it as easy as possible to accomplish the revised strategy until it feels natural. Otherwise, the longstanding habits will rush in to take over.

After 45 minutes of walking and trotting focusing on soft gluteal muscles and leg aids that avoid external rotation at the thigh, Heather exclaims that her hip does not hurt. Usually, she is in pain after only 30 minutes.

Recommended exercises: *Pelvic Bridge and Leg Circles.*

Poor Leg Position Disrupts Balance

Your leg position impacts your balance. Proper leg position forms the classic shoulder-hip (pelvis)-heel line. Ideally, your leg is positioned under your body in such a way that if your horse disappeared, you would land standing upright on the arena floor.

While you are sitting in the saddle, if your leg comes too far in front of your body, which can happen when you use your feet rather than your pelvis as a base of support, you are placed behind the horse's movement (fig. 3.34 A). This position is sometimes called a "chair seat." If this happens at posting trot, you tend to fall heavily in the saddle in the *down* phase and struggle to keep balance in the *up* phase. Depending upon the degree of imbalance, you may then rely upon the reins for stability. As such, your horse gets a "slow down" or "stop" message from you (often followed by a kick, creating quite an unsteady trot and a very confused horse).

This "water ski" position can also happen in down transitions if you push into your stirrups to support your balance. This body position invites

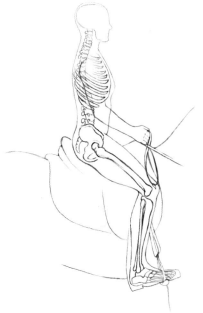

3.34 A *This rider is in a chair-seat position. The legs are too far forward, placing the rider behind the motion of the horse. The rider's spine is often flexed (rounded or C-shaped) with this leg position.*

About Your Body: Sacroiliac Joint Pain

The sacroiliac (SI) joint is the joint between the *sacrum* (the five fused vertebrae that make up the back of the pelvis) and the two *ilia* (the main bones of the pelvis)—see figs. 2.6 and 2.7, p. 28. It is a stress-relieving joint that has minimal movement. Pain can occur at the SI joint with excessive movement or stress. Balanced strength and flexibility of the opposing muscle groups of the hip joint (flexors and extensors, abductors and adductors, and internal and external rotators) can help prevent SI pain. Strain across the joint occurs when the right and left legs pull in different directions, causing a rotational stress across the pelvis (see "The Rider's Challenge" on p. 120). This can happen in the saddle while giving unilateral leg aids or drawing the leg too far back when applying an aid. Work for an anchored pelvic position when using single-leg aids to prevent disruption of pelvic position and strain across the SI joint.

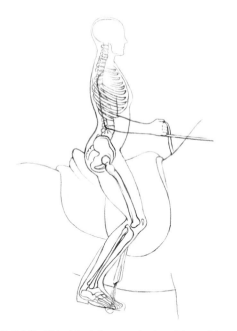

3.34 B *This rider is in a perched position, with too much weight on the front of the pelvic floor. The legs are too far back, pitching the rider forward in an unstable and precarious position. This position is often accompanied by an extended (arched) spine position.*

your horse to fall onto his forehand against the bridle. By keeping your legs underneath your body, you are better able to stay in upright balance over your horse's motion regardless of gait or transition. In this position you can act as a conductor for your horse, proactively influencing his movement from your center rather than reacting to what happens and losing your secure position. And, when you improve *your* balance, you improve *your horse's* balance.

A leg position that is too far forward can also cause you to pitch your torso forward at the hip joint in an effort to balance. This is an inefficient strategy, as the reins are likely to be included in this balance attempt, to the detriment of elastic contact. As well, the posture adopted in this compensatory position is usually extended (arched) with the resulting risk of back strain.

An unsteady leg position that falls behind you also compromises balance (fig. 3.34 B). If your leg is too far back, your body will pitch forward and you'll find yourself in a very precarious position

A Pretty Picture

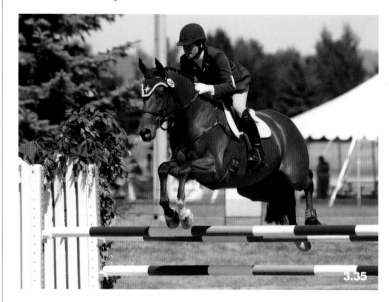

3.35

Meika Descher rides her gelding DeNovo. Meika's leg is correctly positioned underneath the center of her body. This leg position supports her balanced torso over this fence. A leg too far forward would place her behind the horse's motion, and a leg too far back would preclude secure balance. Exercises to help you gain control of leg position include the Pelvic Bridge series; Straight Legs; Ball Tongs; and Knee Folds.

A Pretty Picture

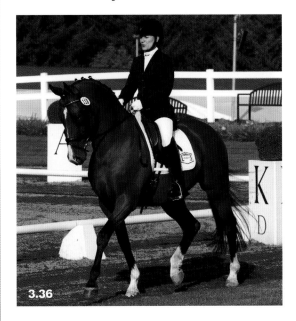

3.36

Paula Helm rides H.S. Whrapsody in a balanced and supple position. Paula reports that Whrapsody can be tense in the show arena, and she has learned that she must keep her legs released and supple to not feed into his anxiety. She gains support from her core muscles for her balance. You can develop this with Abdominal Curls: Crisscross; Spine Extension on Mat; Plank on Mat: Knees or Feet; and Plank on Ball. You develop awareness of your leg muscles with Pelvic Bridge; Knee Circles; Leg Circles; Knee Folds; and Leg Lifts on Ball.

About Your Body: **Arthritis**

Arthritis is inflammation of a joint. While there are many causes of arthritis, including systemic disease, the most common, *osteoarthritis* (degenerative joint disease), results from wear and tear from trauma, overuse, or simply aging.

Arthritis presents with pain in the joint, swelling, and decreased movement. Over time, weakness and stiffness develop. Decreased movement and activity contribute to weight gain, reduced physical fitness, and perhaps depression. The type of arthritis is determined from a careful history and physical exam. Radiographs or other imaging studies may be indicated.

Osteoarthritis comes from progressive damage to the cushioning cartilage of the joints. This interferes with joint function and causes pain. Osteoarthritis typically affects joints that bear weight: knees, hips, and back. Other joints can be affected, particularly if they have been previously injured. Osteoarthritis is more common as we get older; other risk factors include obesity and a sedentary lifestyle. Treatment is directed at preventing the arthritis from getting worse: strengthening the muscles around the joint for support, anti-inflammatory medications, and if relevant, weight loss. In severe cases, joint replacement may be necessary.

Like other musculoskeletal problems, prevention of arthritis in equestrians comes from maintaining fitness and proper body mechanics. Traumatic injuries, unfortunately, do occur around horses. Pay attention and move mindfully to keep your work with them safe. When joint pain occurs, have it evaluated and institute a program to prevent progression.

indeed—one that challenges your ability to keep control of your horse and strips you of your balance tools. In this position, any unexpected movement from your horse can completely unseat you.

Moving on in Balance

Now that you have your legs moving with your horse and more under your control, let's set the same goals for your arms. In the next chapter, we'll explore the anatomy relevant to establishing contact via the reins, as well as further preparing you to rely on your core muscles for maintaining balance.

4 Body Control: Arms

Focus (chapter 1) and support of correct posture (chapter 2) allowed you to learn that your strong legs can be controlled for efficient and effective riding (chapter 3). Now, I'll help you get your arms under control for independent and elastic contact with your horse.

For most of us, much of our day involves thinking, talking, writing, typing, and generally interacting with the world through our eyes and our computer—running our life from the shoulders up. The upper body becomes command central and the arms take on the role of controlling the entire body. Upper-body focus leads to the shoulder muscles, rather than the torso muscles, taking on the job of initiating movement and supporting balance. Since they aren't designed for this job, shoulder pain, neck pain, and headaches can result.

When on horseback, keeping command central in the upper body and shoulders precludes effective riding. The *center* of your body, *not* your upper body, needs to control balance and movement. Without this, you risk managing your horse and your ride using information only from what you see, rather than from what you *feel*. And further, you risk making corrections to your horse only with your hands—via the reins—rather than with your whole body.

Relying on your shoulders and arms for balance causes shoulder tightness and a tendency to lean on the reins for stability.

Balancing from the reins has obvious negative consequences for your horse, as he feels restriction and discomfort from the harsh contact through the bridle. When you correct with the reins only, you risk riding your horse "front to back" and forgetting about the whole horse. Correct rein aids allow, direct, or restrict aspects of your horse's energy and must be delivered with mobility and elasticity, as well as independence between the right and left. Your arms must essentially become part of the bridle, moving with your horse and guiding the energy from him (fig. 4.1, and see fig. 3.1, p. 85). This cannot happen when you are using the reins as handles for balance or when your shoulder tension blocks against the movement of your horse.

A Pretty Picture

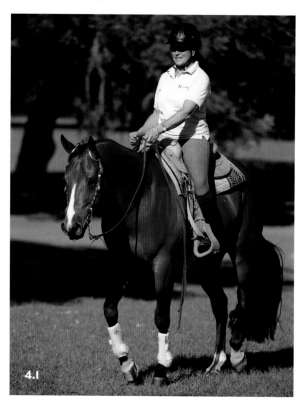

4.1

Lynn Palm shows clear suppleness of her left arm for elastic, steady, and independent contact while riding What About Lark, a 2003 Quarter Horse owned by Ruth Burkhalter. Lynn describes What About Lark as relaxed, and she works to reward his willing nature by staying balanced in her body and "allowing" in her arms. You can see a "giving" feeling in her left arm, offering What About Lark room to move forward. While the amount of contact you have in the reins will vary according to riding discipline, what is common is the requirement for that contact to be consistent and respectful to the horse. You can develop independent rein aids from core stability and control of your arms developed with Hug-a-Tree: Both Arms and Hug-a-Tree: Single Arm.

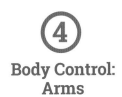

Body Control:
Arms

Anatomy of Arms

Bones

The arms hang off the upper body at the shoulder joint. This joint, like the hip joint, allows a wide range of movement. Via a complex system of muscles, you can move your arms out in front of you, behind you, out to the side, overhead, across your body, and in internal and external rotation. Although few of these actions are desired during riding, keeping the joint mobile and supple avoids rigidity.

Important arm bones include the *humerus* (upper arm bone); the *scapula* (shoulder blade); the *clavicle*; the *ulna* and the *radius* (the bones of the forearm); and the hand, composed of many bones (fig. 4.2). The elbow connects the forearm to the upper arm. It is basically a hinge joint and is well suited to follow the motion of the horse's neck. The wrist allows many movements, including small, refining rein aids. Finally, fingers closed around the reins stabilize rein length.

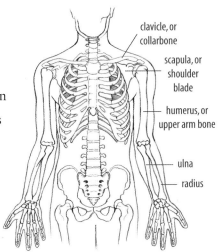

4.2 *The bones of the arm.*

Shoulder Girdle Muscles

The shoulder joint is relatively shallow, compared to the hip joint, so joint stability and alignment depend much more on muscle tone. Figures 4.3 A & B show important shoulder girdle muscles for riding awareness. Imbalance of the strong muscles of the shoulder girdle can easily displace the humerus within the shoulder joint, diminishing range of motion and causing pain.

The *pectoralis major muscle* forms the front part of the armpit. This muscle pulls the shoulder forward. Excess pectoralis major muscle tightness rounds the shoulder and can contribute to a flexed (rounded) posture.

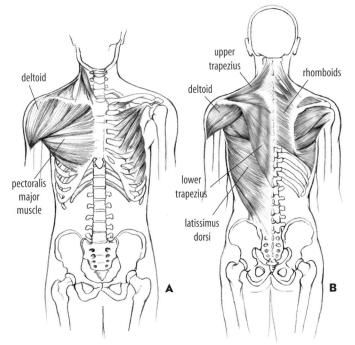

4.3 A & B *The anterior shoulder muscles (A), and the posterior shoulder muscles (B).*

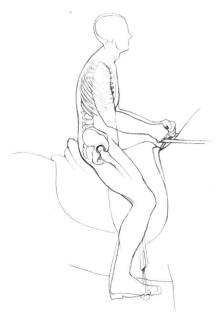

4.4 A *Tight shoulders rounded forward.*

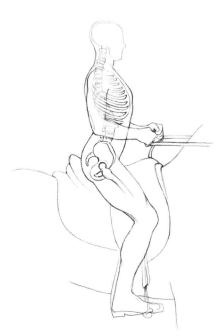

4.4 B *Tight shoulders pulled up and back, creating upper back and arm tension.*

Figure 4.3 B on p. 133 shows the posterior shoulder girdle muscles. The fan-shaped *trapezius* can pull the shoulder up into a shrug or back and down in a more desired position. The *deltoid* forms the upper contour of the shoulder and lifts the arm out to the side.

The *latissimus dorsi muscle* joins the humerus to the whole of the back, thus connecting the arm to the center of the body. This muscle forms the bulk of the back of your armpit. It is one of my favorite muscles for its centering effect. When balanced with appropriate abdominal muscle support to preserve spine alignment, this muscle, along with the lower trapezius, gives the rider great upper-body stability. It connects the arm and shoulder girdle to the center of the body, allowing a secure anchor for supple movement. From this comes an elastic connection that doesn't pull, even when the horse tends to be strong in the bridle.

The *rhomboids*, another important, although smaller, pair of muscles, lie between the medial edge of the scapula and the spine. These muscles assist in pulling the shoulder blades together, and along with the lower trapezius, counteract the unwanted rounding action of the pectoralis major muscle in the front of the shoulder.

Beneath the large and more superficial muscles of the shoulder girdle lies a group of muscles, the *rotator cuff* that facilitates internal and external rotation of the upper arm. Our forward-focused life risks losing strength and function of the posterior portion of the rotator cuff, the external rotators. However, in the context of riding, we need this muscle group to stabilize arm position. Without balance in all the muscles of the shoulder, misalignment, impingement, and overuse strain can result.

Ideally, your arms hang by your sides with your elbows roughly at your waist. Not all riders have the same arm length, however, so elbow position might vary. I encourage a rein length that allows some elbow bend and gives a sense of your hands being out in front of you. Too long of a rein brings your hands back to your abdominal area and restricts their movement. Too short of a rein may result in either pulling or restricting your horse through the bridle, a locked and straight elbow, or a forward position of your torso.

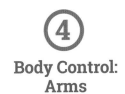
Any fitness program should include arm exercises to develop balanced function of the shoulder girdle and smooth movement at the shoulder without disrupting postural alignment (figs. 4.4 A & B). The result is motion that is efficient and appears fluid and easy, like a ballerina's, but in fact, it requires awareness. The arm exercises selected in this program are designed to develop a strong connection of the arm and shoulder girdle to the torso, allowing the arm to get support and stability from the entire body, and enabling suppleness and elasticity rather than stiffness and grabbing.

EXERCISES to Connect the Arm, Shoulder Girdle, and Torso

Hug-a-Tree: Both Arms

Teaches you that your arms can be mobile about your trunk without disrupting posture, position, or balance.

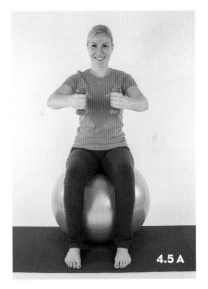

4.5 A

1 Sit upright on an exercise ball, feet flat on the floor, hip-joint width apart.

2 Use free weights (the weight should be challenging but not a struggle—I use 2-pound weights in my classes). Raise your arms in front of you just below shoulder height, with your elbows slightly bent, as if "hugging a tree" (fig. 4.5 A).

3 Take an easy inhale breath, and on the exhale breath open your arms out to the side (fig. 4.5 B). Bring them back in front of you as you inhale.

4 Repeat 6 to 8 times.

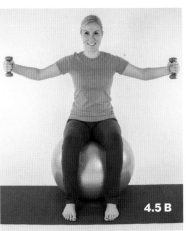

4.5 B

Keep your elbows lifted, but avoid shrugging your shoulders. Keep the bend in your elbow stable throughout the movement. Do not let your arm movement alter your posture. You might feel a tendency to lean back as your arms come in front of you, and to arch your spine and lean forward as your arms go out to the side. Feel your shoulder blades slide together as your arms open out to the side. This might create a beneficial stretch in the pectoralis muscle in the front of your shoulder.

Hug-a-Tree: Single Arm

Improve balance when you move one arm at a time.

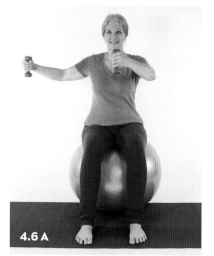

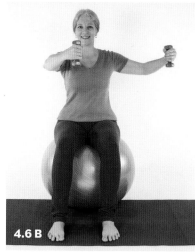

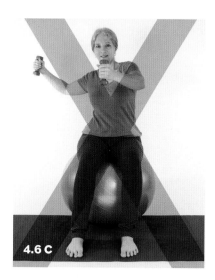

1 Sit upright on an exercise ball, feet flat on the floor, hip-joint width apart.

2 Use free weights (the weight should be challenging but not a struggle—I use 2-pound weights in my classes). Raise your arms in front of you just below shoulder height, with your elbows slightly bent, as if "hugging a tree" (see fig. 4.5 A, p. 135).

3 Take an easy inhale breath, and on the exhale breath stabilize the left side of your body while you reach your right arm out to the side (fig. 4.6 A). Bring your right arm back in front of you as you inhale.

4 On the next exhale breath, stabilize the right side of your body while you reach your left arm out to the side (fig. 4.6 B). Bring your left arm back in front of you as you inhale.

5 Repeat 3 to 4 times for each arm.

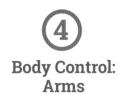

Try to stay upright and steady. You may feel your body try to counterbalance the single arm movement by falling to the opposite side (fig. 4.6 C). Anchoring the opposite side first helps prevent this and develops the skill of staying balanced when giving a single rein aid.

Chest Expansion

Develop a correct shoulders-back position with a stable and supported shoulder girdle, not an extended (arched) spine position.

1 Sit upright on an exercise ball or a chair, feet flat on the floor, hip-joint width apart.

2 Hold a 2-pound free weight in each hand; let your arms hang down by your sides, palms facing behind you (fig. 4.7 A).

3 Take an easy inhale breath, and on the exhale breath, reach your arms back by pulling your shoulder blades together.

4 Keep your arms back, and while breathing normally, turn your head to the right and then to the left (fig. 4.7 B).

5 Return your head and arms to the start position.

6 Repeat 4 to 6 times.

Avoid shrugging your shoulders or pushing your chest out during this exercise. Maintain your abdominal muscle support so your posture stays stable.

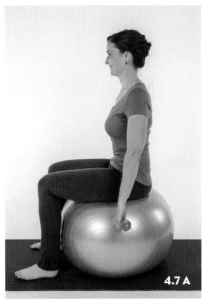

4.7 A

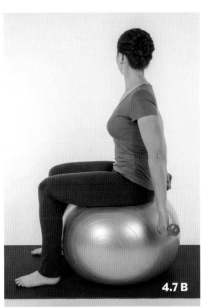

4.7 B

The next two exercises, with a partner, illustrate arm skills useful for riding. I do *not* advise that you always ride in either of the extreme manners illustrated in these exercises. They are meant to define a spectrum of arm mobility and stability. I *do* believe that you need these skills for good riding. These exercises are described using exercise balls; you can also do them standing.

Partner Arm Suppleness

Feel how supple and moveable your arms can be.

You need a partner, two exercise balls, and two stretch bands.

1 Sit on an exercise ball facing your partner, who also sits on an exercise ball.

2 Grasp the ends of the stretch bands as if holding reins (fig. 4.8 A).

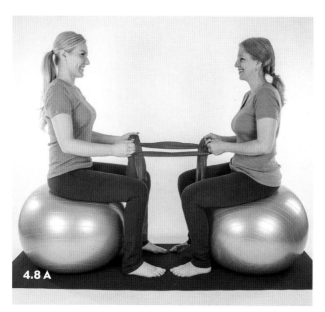

4.8 A

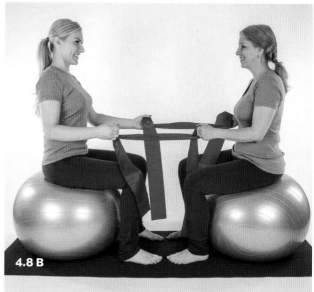

4.8 B

3 Alternate roles: First, one of you is "horse" and the other is "rider." Have enough contact between the two of you to create slight tension in the stretch band "reins."

4 When you are "horse," move your arms back and forth, not necessarily rhythmically; some randomness is good.

5 When you are "rider," keep steady contact with your horse partner by moving your arms while she moves her arms (fig. 4.8 B). The effect should be even pressure in your reins throughout.

6 After a few moments, reverse roles.

Keep the movements slow so steadiness is possible. Feel how you can nearly predict how your "horse partner" will move her arms, using your focus and balance. Avoid shrugging your shoulders; keep correct posture. Feel the potential for mobility and elasticity in your arms.

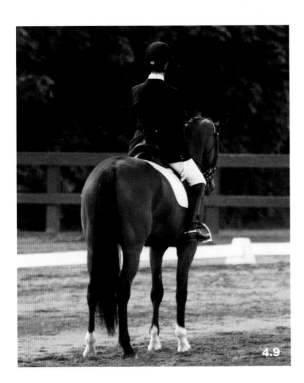

4.9

DG and I are at a halt in 2011. Even though my shoulder blades wing out a bit from my upper back, they are suitably positioned and stabilized. This stable arm position makes it clear to DG that we are no longer moving. As we move off in trot, my rein connection will soften to allow her to move forward. Chest Expansion and Partner Arm Stability are exercises to develop a correct "shoulders back" position.

Partner Arm Stability

Develop body-position stability in order to prevent a "pulling" horse from unseating you.

For this exercise you need a partner, two exercise balls, and two stretch bands.

1 Sit on an exercise ball facing your partner, who also sits on an exercise ball.

2 Grasp the ends of the stretch bands as if holding reins (fig. 4.10 A).

3 Alternate roles: First, one of you is "horse" and the other is "rider." Have enough contact between the two of you to create slight tension in the stretch band "reins."

4 When you are "horse" (the person on the left in fig. 4.10 B), gradually increase tension in the band so you are pulling against your rider.

5 If you are "rider" (the person on right in fig. 4.10 B), keep a steady body position despite your "horse's" pulling.

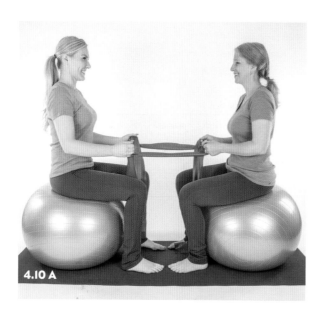

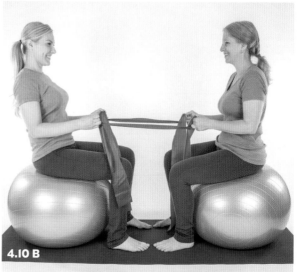

6 After a few moments, reverse roles.

When you are the rider, prepare for the pulling horse by feeling your arms anchor down your back: Think of the V-like lower trapezius and latissimus dorsi muscles. Keep your elbows securely by your sides. Stabilize your balance by engaging your abdominal muscles. As your "horse partner" pulls, feel how you can exactly mirror the pulling force by engaging the shoulder girdle and core muscles, so that you are not moved or put off balance by your pulling horse partner. Use an exhale breath to anchor and stabilize your body. Avoid actively pulling against your horse partner; just try to match the pulling force. This allows you to soften and "reward" your partner when she stops the pulling. If you actively pull, when your partner releases you will fall backward out of balance, tugging on your partner. If you are the "horse," don't be too sudden or strong—you want this exercise to be productive, not harsh.

About Your Body:
Shoulder Impingement

The *humerus* (upper arm bone) rests in a very shallow joint space to form the shoulder joint. While this configuration allows a large range of motion, it makes it relatively easy for the humerus to become misaligned within the joint. Many muscles, superficial and deep, influence the movement and placement of the humerus. Lack of balanced tone and flexibility of the shoulder-girdle musculature can lead to misalignment. A common imbalance is weakening of the external rotators, which allows the head of the humerus to shift forward and upward, decreasing the joint space. When this happens, some arm movement, such as reaching overhead, causes the humerus to compress sensitive tendons and bursae in the shoulder joint, thus causing pain and limited range of motion. This is called *shoulder impingement syndrome*.

Riders are at risk of shoulder impingement from poor shoulder mechanics, both while riding, as well as work on the ground. Rounded shoulders, and shoulders pulled forward with elbows sticking out to the side (internal rotation), are common unbalanced arm positions while riding. The same arm positions are equally harmful when doing barn work. The muscle imbalance risks pulling the humerus forward in the shoulder joint and contributing to shoulder impingement syndrome.

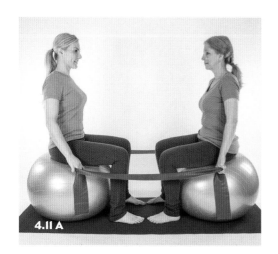

4.11 A

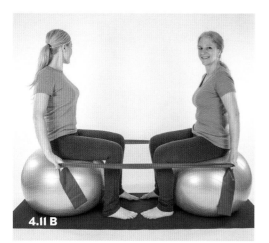

4.11 B

Partner Chest Expansion

In addition to stretching your shoulders back, this exercise improves your sense of contact.

For this exercise you need a partner, two exercise balls, and two stretch bands.

1 Sit on an exercise ball facing your partner, who also sits on an exercise ball.

2 Grasp the ends of the stretch bands holding your arms straight down by your sides with palms facing behind you (fig. 4.11 A). Keep enough tension in the stretch band "reins" so that there isn't any slack between the two of you.

3 Perform the Chest Expansion exercise together. Take an easy inhale breath, and on the exhale breath, press both arms behind you and pull your shoulder blades together.

4 Hold your arms back and turn your head to the right, and then to the left, and then release your arms forward (fig. 4.11 B).

5 Repeat 4 to 6 times.

Work to match your partner's effort to keep an even excursion of your arms and your partner's arms. Try to elastically begin and end the movement, tuning in to your partner's movement. It helps if one of you calls out the movement, so you can predict when to start. Avoid pushing your abdomen out in front of you as you press your arms back. Keep your alignment stable and upright.

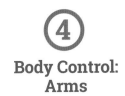

Shoulder Stretch
Combat tightness in the muscles of the shoulder girdle.

You can do this stretch either sitting on an exercise ball or standing.

1 Grasp an elastic stretch band or a towel with both hands shoulder-width apart, or farther (fig. 4.12 A).

2 Reach over and behind your head with the band taut in order to stretch your shoulders back (fig. 4.12 B). You should feel the stretch in the muscle of the front of your armpit (the pectoralis major muscle).

3 Adjust the stretch band or towel tension so that you can comfortably lift your arms over your head and behind your back.

4 Repeat the stretch 3 to 4 times.

Avoid pressing your abdomen forward or arching your spine as your arms reach overhead and then behind you. Keep your weight balanced over both feet.

The pectoralis major muscle is often tight in people whose lives involve a great deal of desk or computer work. This stretch promotes a correct shoulder position and posture on and off the horse.

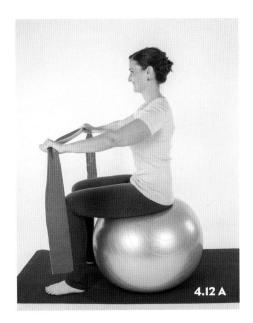

4.12 A

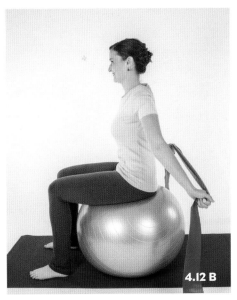

4.12 B

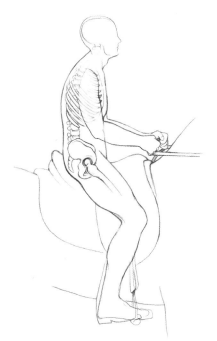

4.13 *A shoulder that is rounded forward contributes to a flexed (rounded or C-shaped) posture.*

Common Arm Position and Function Challenges

Like the muscles of the hip joint, the muscles of the shoulder girdle can have important effects on posture. As mentioned, a rider with a computer-based desk job can suffer from a chronically flexed (rounded, C-shaped) posture—both from sitting all day without proper spine support and from constant frontward use of the arms, causing tight pectoral muscles (fig. 4.13). This postural problem is common. If this describes your work environment, remember to get up now and then to stretch, move, and restore good alignment.

It is very important that this rounded shoulder and flexed posture be corrected precisely. Improving this position requires adjusting the position of the shoulder girdle around the rib cage, as well as restoring the normal lumbar curve of the spine. It is common that this position is changed incorrectly by only leaning the upper body back. The shoulders remain rounded forward, but the lumbar spine is changed too much into an arch, or spine extension. The strong pectoralis major muscle resists adjusting the position of the shoulder girdle, and instead the movement is shifted to the vulnerable and more moveable spine (see The Rider's Challenge: "Rounded Shoulders," p. 145).

This takes one problem (rounded shoulders) and creates two problems (rounded shoulders and an arched spine). This evasion of the rider's body can result in an undesired S-shaped posture (see p. 61). It is important to recognize that shoulder and postural issues need to be addressed individually. Adjust spine alignment and then shoulder alignment. Remember that the shoulder girdle can move around the rib cage independently of movement of the spine (even though it may not want to). The *Chest Expansion* exercise helps clarify this movement.

Because of the shallow shoulder joint, improper arm and shoulder alignment while riding can cause injury (see "Shoulder Impingement," p. 141). If you are dealing with a horse that tends to pull, be vigilant about arm support during your training. A common strategy for power from the arms while riding is pulling the shoulders forward and rotating the elbows away from the body.

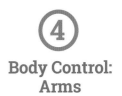

Rounded Shoulders

Laurie expresses concern that her lack of stable balance is interfering with the development of her young horse. Laurie is a veteran rider who has explored many disciplines. She recently gravitated to dressage and rides a five-year-old, 16-hand, Dutch Warmblood gelding, named Mitch. Laurie describes herself as motivated and ambitious, perhaps too much so. And she describes Mitch as mellow.

Laurie warms up at working trot. Mitch's trot lacks activity. Laurie works to keep his trot tempo active by thrusting her body forward at the top of the rise while posting; her gaze drifts downward, her shoulders and upper body round forward, her elbows move away from her sides, and her hands turn in toward her abdomen.

At the halt, I show Laurie a better upper-body alignment. However, she struggles to make the appropriate adjustments. When asked to bring her shoulder blades together—stretching her pectoralis muscle—her shoulders lock, and her lower back arches. This is a common "evasion" in riders with this problem. The shoulders, tight and pulled forward, resist changing position and stretching. From the body's standpoint, it is easier to shift the whole upper body back and arch the lumbar spine than to just move the shoulders around the rib cage. In an attempt to correct a rounded posture from tight shoulders, the S-shaped posture can result (see p. 61).

Remedy

To help Laurie sort out this issue, I encourage her to think of her shoulders connecting down her back in a V shape (following the latissimus dorsi muscle-fiber alignment—see fig. 4.3 B, p. 133). At the same time, to avoid an arched spine, I have her feel her rib cage in front remain stable and connected to the pelvis by her abdominal muscles. I describe the upper-body and lower-body planes used in the S-posture correction (see fig. 2.44, p. 65).

Laurie struggles with this new position, but determination is on her side. Back at trot, this more upright posture allows her to feel her horse's effort at impulsion, rather than block his energy. There is improved freedom at her hip joint. Her contact through the bridle improves and is more sensitive, as her arm muscles are more supple in this balanced position. She can feel Mitch's energy come from his hindquarters and flow through her body at the back of her upper thigh, and out in front of her (see fig. 2.2, p. 25). These subtle but real changes improve Mitch's gait quality and give Laurie a better sense of riding "back to front."

Exercises for Laurie: *Spine Extension on Mat; Spine Extension: Scarecrow; Hug-a-Tree: Both Arms; Shoulder Stretch.*

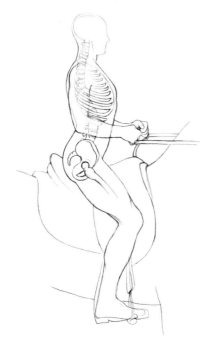

4.14 *A shoulder that is tense and lifted up toward the rider's ears contributes to an extended (arched) posture.*

This employs the strong anterior shoulder muscle, the pectoralis major, and places the arms in internal rotation to support against a pulling horse. However, this strategy risks shoulder strain from unbalanced forces. A more effective strategy is to anchor the elbows by your sides, and gain support from the muscles of the posterior shoulder girdle: the lattisimus dorsi, lower trapezius, and external rotators. Correct stability with these muscles connects your arms down your back; these muscles form the back of your armpit and anchor your shoulder. Matched with your stabilizing core muscles, this system supports your arms in better alignment for less strain and more effectiveness.

Riders who carry work and life stresses in their shoulders can end up with a chronic "shoulder shrug" and extreme tension in the upper body. This muscle tension pulls them up and away from their center of gravity, into an extended (arched) posture (fig. 4.14). They may experience pain in the mid back because this region is overworking.

RIDER'S CHALLENGE

Upper Body Tension

Cassie comes to my Pilates-based, small-group exercise classes. She is new to dressage and is thrilled to have a talented Warmblood gelding, Sam, who is patient with her learning. She explains that her trainer sent her to my classes to improve her shoulders.

"She always nags at me to relax my shoulders. For some reason this is really hard for me to do," Cassie says.

In class, I note that when an exercise requires arm movement, she initiates it by first pulling her shoulders up to her ears. My challenge is to teach Cassie how to move her arms without this obligatory shrug and to help her feel balanced from her torso.

Months later, Cassie comes for a riding lesson. A tall woman with a longish torso, Cassie looks drawn away from her horse with negative tension and energy in her upper body and shoulders. She holds her spine in a rigid arch, with her seat bones pointing behind her. She draws her legs slightly forward and holds the reins tight as she pilots her horse around the arena by pulling on one rein and then the other, her legs giving a random kick every now and then. She relies on her arms and shoulders to do most of the work.

Remedy

My goal is to get Cassie feeling the tools of stability within her torso for balance in the saddle. First, we work on breathing to help her get anchored in the saddle and define the pelvis, not the shoulder girdle, as her base of support.

A Pretty Picture

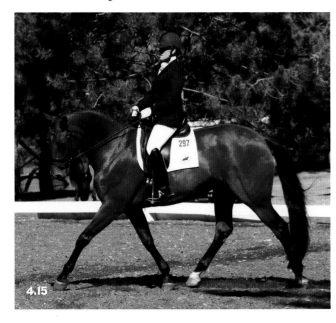

4.15

Lisa Boyer has an elastic contact with Zamora consistent with a supple, not tense, shoulder. Zamora is a very willing horse and Lisa is always striving to be soft with her rein aids. Lisa can be this sensitive rider because she stays stable in her posture and balance. From her steady body position, Lisa can make subtle adjustments with her reins through the ride. Exercises to help develop body stability and arm mobility include: Plank on Mat: Knees; Plank on Mat: Feet; Plank on Ball; Quadruped: Single; Quadruped: Diagonal; Hug-a-Tree: Both Arms; Hug-a-Tree: Single Arm. A great exercise to develop this stability with elasticity is Partner Arm Stability.

"But I feel like I'm slouching!" Cassie protests as I guide her pelvis slightly back in the saddle to a more neutral position. But when she looks in the mirror she sees how a small change in the position of her pelvis settles her down into the saddle—a very new feeling for her—and contributes to a sense of being connected to her horse's body, not perched on top.

I urge Cassie to focus on her core muscles, feeling a constant hum of connection to these muscles and teaching her brain that they are "there" to support her position and balance in the saddle. Back on the rail at walk, I coach Cassie to keep the inward stabilizing abdominal muscles in her awareness. When she does this, I see her release her shoulder tension. She no longer grips the reins like handles, and her contact becomes more elastic and following. Sam responds by lowering his usually inverted neck and reaching to the bit. Confused by the feeling of slouching, Cassie often looks in the mirror to confirm that this changed position is not sloppy. She begins to feel that releasing her shoulders helps her "sit deep," something she had been told to do but didn't know how.

My next client arrives outside the arena, prompting Sam to lift his head suddenly. Cassie responds by reverting to her shoulder-focused control and grabbing the reins. But a centered breath reminds her to release her shoulder tension and sit back down in the saddle.

Exercises for Cassie: *Rib Cage Breathing 1 and 2; Pelvic Rocking: Supine; Pelvic Rocking on Ball: Front to Back; Abdominal Curls; Leg Lifts on Ball; Shoulder Stretch.*

Balance and integration of the body for effective riding is difficult with tight shoulders. It is tempting to view tight shoulders as an isolated problem that you can solve by just bringing your shoulders down. Unfortunately, if you follow this cue without a sense of your center, you risk further pulling away from your source of stable balance (your torso), and focusing too much on your arms as the problem (it is most likely your core that is failing). If this describes you, find your center and allow your shoulders to do less work. But be warned: When you correct this posture, you will probably feel that you are leaning or rounding forward. Remember that what is correct does not feel normal until it becomes a habit. But improving your efficiency of balance and position, as well as gaining support from all the torso muscles (not just those of the mid back), will convince you that the change is a good one.

Novice or fearful riders often overwork the shrugging muscles (upper trapezius, among others) as their body tries to find some sense of security in the foreign place of being on horseback. This rider must develop a sense of being anchored to the saddle through the pelvis to release the tight shoulder girdle. This problem of self-confidence in the saddle is one particularly amenable to off-horse work. The improved sense of self and trust in your body gained from improved strength and awareness not only supplies you with concrete tools for stability in the saddle, but also diminishes fear.

Arms Must Function Independently

Use of your arms for a rein aid must not disrupt your posture, alignment, and balance. This is challenging: In the saddle, your upper body can be relatively mobile, making it easy to lean in one direction or the other to counterbalance a rein aid. (Think of your body's response to the *Hug-a-Tree: Single Arm* exercise, p. 136.) But leaning causes an unwanted shift in your weight—confusing your horse. Stability of position starts with balancing from the muscles of your torso. Arm suppleness, mobility, and control are then possible.

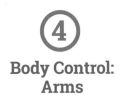
RIDER'S CHALLENGE |||||||||||||||||||||||||||||||||||||||||||||||||||||||||||||||||||||||||||||||||||||||||

Shoulder Tension Causes Arm Numbness

Tiffany contacts me interested in improving her core strength and body control for riding. She has just finished a course of physical therapy for bulging discs in her neck that were causing numbness in her arms from nerve compression. During therapy, she avoided riding. She is anxious to ride again, but a few attempts have resulted in arm numbness. We start with off-horse exercises in my studio, with the goal of evaluating her riding after a few sessions.

Remedy

My focus in the studio is to help Tiffany find secure balance from her core muscles, improve her awareness of how her shoulders tensed during *any* exercise (especially if it requires lots of focus), and how to rewire that habitual response. We work on *Rib Cage Breathing* as a preparation for every exercise, including in the preparation of a conscious release of her shoulders.

I tell her, "As you exhale, release the tension in your shoulders, and send that energy to your core, or abdominal and back muscles."

After several sessions in the studio, Tiffany comes for a riding lesson. It is immediately obvious why riding brings on her arm numbness. Every time she rides a transition or her horse takes an odd step or startles, Tiffany grabs the reins and pulls her shoulders up toward her ears, and her body is pulled forward. This "shrugging" muscle tension adds pressure to nerve roots already impinged by her cervical-disc problem, and her arms become numb.

We go back to basics. We stay at walk and practice breathing in the same manner as in the studio. I coach her to, "Take an easy breath in, and as you breathe out, release shoulder tension and put positive tension in the muscles of your core. Use the breath as your half-halt. Use your breath to steady yourself in the saddle when your horse startles. Brainwash yourself to have your stress response be in your core, not your shoulders."

This is a huge challenge for Tiffany. But she has the motivation of avoiding her symptoms to encourage her to make this positive change.

Most riders know that resorting to the shoulders and reins for balance and stability is counter to effective riding. For riders like Tiffany, it is not just about being effective, it is also about avoiding harm to her body.

Exercises: *Rib Cage Breathing 1 and 2; Pelvic Rocking: Front to Back; and Pelvic Rocking: Side to Side.*

Arm Control Facilitates Training

If you need to use more rein as a restraining aid for a strong horse, be careful that your torso position stays solid upright on the vertical in neutral spine alignment. It is tempting to lean back, press your feet forward, and use body weight to control your horse. This works in the short term and is appropriate for a bolting horse. But to improve your horse's balance, leaning back is the worst thing to do. Leaning back puts you behind the horse's movement and gives the horse something to lean against.

When you lack suitable stability, a strong horse can pull you forward, putting you in a dysfunctional position—perched forward out of the saddle without a base of support—and opening the door to the horse for more evasions. If your horse gets strong, find your base of support by anchoring your pelvis to the saddle with your core muscles and anchoring your upper arms by your sides (think of those latissimus dorsi muscles).

A Pretty Picture

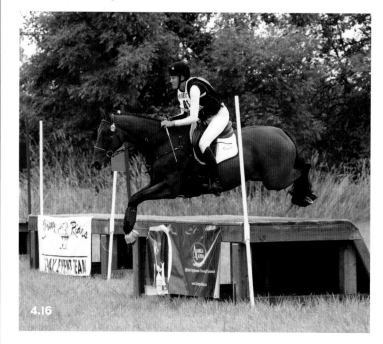

4.16

Patience O'Neal shows clear independence in her arms to allow the 2002 Thoroughbred gelding Markus freedom in his neck over this cross-country fence. Note that the center of her body is in the middle of the horse, and her legs are underneath her body, supporting balance. As a result her arms remain elastic and "allowing." You can develop independent arm function by strengthening your core (Plank on Mat: Knees; Plank on Mat: Feet; Plank on Ball; Quadruped: Single; Quadruped: Diagonal) and gaining control of arm position (Hug-a-Tree: Both Arms; Hug-a-Tree: Single Arm; Chest Expansion; Partner Arm Suppleness; Partner Arm Stability; Partner Chest Expansion).

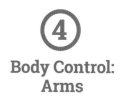

RIDER'S CHALLENGE ||||||||||||||||||||||||||||||||||||||||||||||||||||||||||||||||||||||||||||||||||||||||||||||||

Rein Aid Disrupts Balance

"I am having so much trouble maintaining bend in the left-lead canter," Jeff announces as we start the lesson on his 10-year-old Thoroughbred gelding, Gregor.

I watch Jeff and Gregor warm up at working trot and canter on the right lead. Jeff's posture is fairly good to the right, although he tends to muscle the horse around with his strong legs, rather than follow Gregor's movement. I note that Jeff struggles to control Gregor's right, or outside, shoulder when they trot left. Jeff is "left-sided" and sits to the right as they trot left, overbending Gregor's neck to the inside.

At the left-lead canter, Gregor braces against the left rein; Jeff pulls more and falls more to the right. Gregor also falls more and more to his right and eventually stumbles into a hollow, running, unbalanced trot.

Jeff's lateral-balance problem is made worse when he uses his left rein. Using his left arm increases tone in his left side and sends him more and more to the right. The more he uses his left rein, the worse his balance gets, until Gregor falls apart. My first goal is to help Jeff feel balanced in the middle of the saddle.

Remedy

I have Jeff do small pelvic side-rocking movements in the saddle. Not surprisingly, he finds it easy to lift the left side of his pelvis, but challenging to lift the right. While I hold the reins, he practices small spine-twist movements, keeping his seat bones evenly weighted as he turns his upper body. When rotating left, he falls right: I have him lift his right seat bone a bit as he turns left with his shoulders—this helps his balance. While his rightward rotation is initially restricted, it is easier for him to rotate to the right when he keeps even weight over his seat bones.

Back on the rail, I have Jeff do some sitting trot figures of eight to help him feel centered going both directions. Rotating his shoulders slightly to the right, or to the outside of the circle, helps Jeff stay "in the middle" when tracking to the left (rather than falling right). While the change feels extreme to him, it is really a simple correction: He stops twisting his body too far to the left. Thinking of turning right keeps his shoulders appropriately aligned with Gregor's shoulders and brings his weight to a more centered position.

At left-lead canter, I again coach Jeff to slightly rotate his body to the right. I urge him to avoid using the left rein in such a way that overbends Gregor's neck left, even if this means Gregor is counterbent for the time being. I also give Jeff my "elbow spur" image for his right elbow (see p. 77) and have him turn by bringing his right side to the left. My goal is first for Jeff to feel what it means to not fall right while cantering left. When this position feels secure, he can add the bending aids. Until then, however, Jeff's attempts at bending Gregor with his overbearing left rein cause postural problems in Jeff and straightness issues in Gregor.

While it feels awkward for Jeff to engage the right side of his body while going left, the result in Gregor is profound. With his body closer to being straight, he turns left without falling right and maintains the canter on the 20-meter circle.

Exercises for Jeff: *Pelvic Rocking on Ball: Side to Side; Spine Twist on Ball; Leg Lifts on Ball; Hug-a-Tree: Single Arm.*

From this position your rein aids are functional and are more likely to make positive changes in your horse. I am not suggesting that you ride around and around with your horse hanging on the reins, but if you let your horse change your position, you have lost effectiveness. Work to keep a stable position when your horse pulls; meanwhile, do exercises and transitions geared toward improving your horse's balance.

Some trainers coach riders, "Keep your hands still!" But this cue can be confusing. Your hands *should* move sometimes, depending upon your horse's gait (see chapter 5). *Steady* is a better word to describe hand position: You

A Pretty Picture

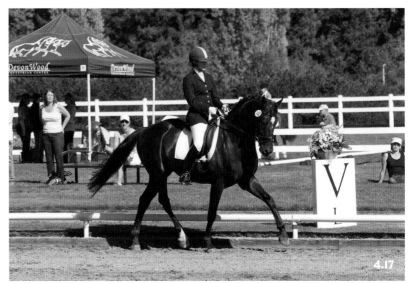

4.17

Catherine Reid has a steady hand position in shoulder-in right with Skywalker HW, and avoids a change in her centered position while applying right-bending aids For some riders, asking for right bend results in a change in body position. A rider can fall left as she asks for her horse to bend right with her right leg. This encourages the horse to fall onto his left shoulder out of balance—and this is made worse if the rider uses too much right rein. True independence of rein and leg aids means that there is no change in the centered position of your pelvis in the middle of the saddle, whether or not you are applying your right leg, left leg, right rein, or left rein. Solid balance with truly independent aids is practiced in Hug-A-Tree: Single Arm and Leg Lifts on Ball.

control where your hands are at all times. Think of it this way: If you had a pressure meter between the reins and your fingers, the pressure would stay quite stable. Clearly, your horse has some role in this goal! And so do you. Keeping your hands steady develops a quiet connection (fig. 4.17).

Arm position can reveal balance problems. An arm that persistently "feels" compelled to cross over your horse's neck is likely adapting for a problem with your body's balance and alignment. If you sit heavily to the left when tracking right, you may find the need to cross your left (outside) hand over your horse's neck to try and control his bulging left shoulder. This arm position is not desirable. Notice what your arm is doing and check your alignment, balance, and position. If you sit heavily to the left while tracking left, you might find your left arm trying to "hold up" your horse's left shoulder by coming up and in, crossing over your horse's neck. Again, note this faulty arm position, and realize it reflects a balance issue. Work to sort out your balance so your arms stay in a correct position.

Your hands and arms must not be dead weight on your horse's mouth; rather, you must keep your arms in self-carriage, just like the rest of you. Otherwise, your horse will feel backward pressure on the reins. To keep a sense of your arms being "alive," imagine a current running through a loop defined as follows: from the bit in your horse's mouth, to the right rein, to your hand holding the right rein, to your right wrist, forearm, elbow, and upper arm, then across your upper back and down the left upper arm, elbow, forearm, wrist, hand, left rein, and back to the bit in your horse's mouth. This loop of current must remain unblocked. Unnecessary tension in any part of your arm, such as from a cocked wrist, a locked elbow, or a shoulder shrug, will block current through this loop, and elasticity will be lost.

Do not equate soft and elastic contact with loose fingers on the reins. Loose fingers allow the reins to easily slip out of your hands, causing you to lose steadiness in the contact. Keep your fingers closed on the reins, making your arm "part of the bridle." Elasticity and soft contact comes from suppleness in your whole arm, not just in your fingers. Certainly your horse feels an increase in squeeze on the rein: just be sure you do not let go of the squeeze so much that you let go of the reins!

Movement at your elbow is key to maintaining a steady contact with your horse's mouth, especially in the walk and canter, in which your horse's neck undulates as part of the mechanic of the gaits. To keep steady contact, you must allow movement of your elbow joints, as well as your shoulders, so that your hands move with your horse's mouth. At the trot, however, your horse's head and neck are quite steady, while his body (and your body) moves up and down. At this gait, your elbows must allow your body to move up and down while your hands stay steady; your hands should *not* go up and down (see chapter 5, p. 165).

A simple example demonstrates the importance of arm-muscle suppleness in preserving elastic contact: Hold a cup of liquid in your right hand and walk around. The liquid will not slosh around much because your supple arm adapts for the movement of your walk to keep the cup level. Now tuck something under your right upper arm and walk around. You will see the liquid slosh

RIDER'S CHALLENGE ||||||||||||||||||||||||||||||||||||||||||||||||||||||||||||||||||||||||||||||||||||||||||||||

Locked Elbows

Jessica trots over after her warm-up with clear frustration on her face.

"He is always looking away with his head up, totally ignoring me," she says. And to prove her point, this eight-year-old Morgan gelding, Lambo, looks left and whinnies.

Jessica and Lambo walk off. Lambo's walk is tense and quick, with a lateral tendency. He is above the bit, and his well-developed, under-neck muscles suggest that this is how he usually moves. Jessica responds to his high-headed posture by pushing her hands down so far that her elbows straighten and her wrists lock. Lambo slows a bit, but his head remains high. A quick kick from Jessica quickens his pace but worsens his tension and walk rhythm.

Jessica is willing to see what happens when she lets go of the reins. Lambo stretches his head out and down, and his walk rhythm improves.

I explain to Jessica that her arm position contributes to Lambo's inverted posture. It may seem like a good idea to put your hands down when your horse puts his head up, but, in fact, it only makes your horse's inverted posture worse!

Remedy

While I hold the reins with one hand, with my other hand I place Jessica's arm in the correct position for a steady contact with Lambo. I then move her arm forward (toward the bit) and back (away from the bit) but always on a line straight to the bit, showing how her arm should move with Lambo's neck. When she shoves her hands

A Pretty Picture

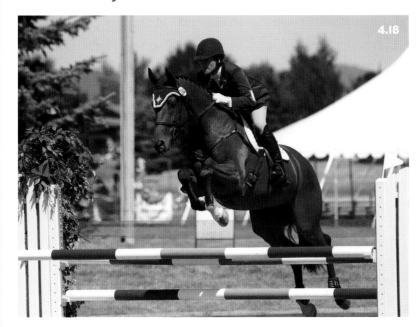

4.18

Meika Descher rides DeNovo (aka "Dino") with her center of balance precisely over that of her horse. Her balance results from control of her torso position from core muscles, as well as a stable leg position underneath her center. From this position, her arms are free to allow Dino's neck to lengthen over the top of the fence. You can develop this independence in your arms and shoulders from Hug-a-Tree: Both Arms; Hug-a-Tree: Single Arm; Partner Arm Stability; and Chest Expansion.

down, it is impossible to have a pleasant connection with Lambo through the bridle. Certainly Lambo has his own issues, but Jessica's job (as the thinking member of the horse-rider team) is to avoid contributing to his issues and then trying to sort them out.

Back at the rail at walk, Jessica rides on a longish rein. I coach her to slowly take up contact, little by little. When she gets close to having some contact, Lambo begins to tense. I have her guide Lambo on a circle line and avoid pressing her arm down, but feel it move back and forth with his head and neck movement. He softens a bit to the slight contact. His tempo slows somewhat, but I urge Jessica to not make a big deal about it right now. Our goal is to improve the harmony between horse and rider. I want Jessica to feel how her stiffness is preventing Lambo from moving freely.

We go back and forth from walking on a long rein to gradually taking up contact on a bending line going both directions, with Jessica fighting her habit of pushing her arms and hands down in a locked position whenever Lambo's head comes up. I encourage her to continue staying with Lambo's head and neck movement by moving her arms back and forth. Over time, Lambo becomes less worried about her taking up the reins, and he responds with less tension. Jessica begins to feel how the rhythm of his walk informs the movement of her arms to stay with his head and neck so contact is more sympathetic.

Exercises for Jessica: *Rib Cage Breathing 1 and 2; Leg Lifts on Ball; Partner Arm Suppleness; Hug-a-Tree: Both Arms and Single Arm.*

around madly as your locked upper arm and elbow can no longer move. (I discovered this while carrying the morning paper under my arm with a cup of coffee in my hand.)

Wrist suppleness allows you to fine-tune your connection with your horse when giving aids. With correct arm position and elbows close to your sides, position your hands with thumbs on top, pointing slightly toward each other, with your wrist joint straight. For subtle rein aids, move your wrist by flexing it or bending it inward. Return to start position after each aid.

With focus, balance from posture, and postural support, and control of your "muscle-men" legs and controlling arms, it is now time to consider your horse. Next I'll explore how you should move with your horse at each gait and transition to promote balance and harmony.

A Pretty Picture

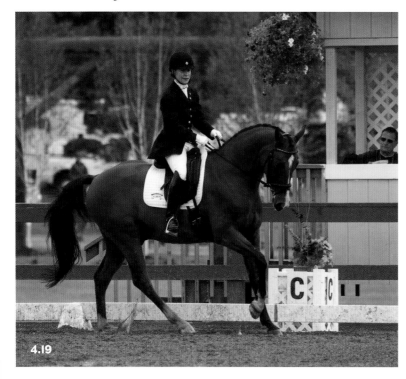

4.19

Paula Helm shows clear independence of her rein aids at canter with H.S. Whrapsody. Looking at her bent elbows, you can sense that she will allow the motion of Whrapsody's head and neck in canter. While I might encourage her to sit back slightly, she is still in very good balance and does not interfere with Whrapsody. Her independent arms result from a stable core and suppleness in the muscles of her shoulder. Exercises that can improve your shoulder suppleness and help develop independent rein aids include Hug-a-Tree, and Partner Arm Suppleness.

5 Understanding Movement

The fifth and final Rider Fundamental considers the basic characteristics of your horse's gaits and how your body moves with each gait. A simple understanding of your horse's gaits is necessary for you to positively influence your horse's movement. In this chapter, I'll review the three gaits—walk, trot, and canter—and for each gait you'll learn "what moves and what shouldn't move much" in your body. You'll be putting your skills of Mental Focus, Proper Posture, and Leg and Arm Control to use! Finally, I will cover strategies for improving balance and using your body efficiently and effectively in transitions and lateral movements.

Consideration of how the horse moves opens the door to riding in harmony. Without considering the character of the horse's gaits, you have no basis from which to improve the horse's way of going. The horse's character of movement is his raw material for you to work with. You must understand how you interact with this material before expecting it to change.

The ability to move in harmonious communication with your horse is the same as riding with "feel." Some say feel is a skill you either have or you don't: If you are lucky to be a rider with feel, you are admired. If, however, you are told you lack this skill, it seems you are doomed to a riding career of struggles. I strongly disagree with this sentiment. While some riders do seem to have a knack for moving naturally with their horse, I wholeheartedly believe you can develop feel in your riding if your position and balance are solid as guided by the Rider Fundamentals.

A rider with feel predicts and interacts with the horse's movements and behaviors as if she can read the horse's mind and body. A rider with feel always appears *with* the horse despite challenges or evasions from the horse. This rider seems to always know just the right amount, and timing of, encouraging or correcting rein or leg aids, and seems to be sitting *inside* the horse, rather than on top. The resulting picture, to the uneducated eye, looks as if the rider is doing nothing (but we know otherwise).

Young riders have a particular knack for feel. With relatively little guidance, a skilled young rider develops the ability to move with the horse and influence

A Pretty Picture

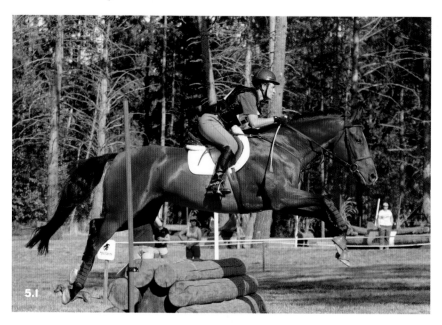

Martha Wehling rides her 2002 Oldenburg/Hanoverian gelding Cavalier (aka "Charlie") in good form over this cross-country fence. She has all the Rider Fundamentals working for her: she is focused on what is ahead, her correct posture keeps her balanced with Charlie, her legs are underneath her providing support, her arms allow freedom for Charlie's head and neck, and she is prepared for Charlie's jump.

him in a positive way. This is not surprising, as learning new movement skills comes naturally at a young age. As we get older, it becomes harder and harder for the brain and body to learn new tasks and make logical choices for balance and coordination. It is not that we can't learn something new; it just takes longer and requires a greater commitment. If you are an older rider and think you lack feel, don't give up. I strongly believe it can be learned and developed.

The tools provided in the Rider Fundamentals are what you need to develop feel. First, a *proactive and attentive mindset* allows you to precisely sense your horse's deviations from the desired character of a gait, movement, or transition (chapter 1). *Balance* (chapter 2) and *body control* (chapters 3 and 4) give you the tools to avoid interfering with your horse's movement. Finally, in this chapter, *learning and understanding your horse's rhythm and movement at each gait*, and how you, the rider, should move with them puts you and your horse on the same page, and the door is open to ride with feel (fig. 5.1).

EXERCISES to Develop Independent Movement

The following exercises expand on *Bounce in Rhythm 1*, from chapter 1. You will bounce in rhythm with a metronome on your ball, further practicing your ability to stay in a steady tempo. Then, you'll be adding coordinated movements of the rest of your body. Just like when you ride, you'll need to keep steady in your rhythm and coordinated in your body movements. These exercises develop independent movement of arms, legs, and torso, and the addition of bouncing adds the background of ongoing movement energy that you experience in the saddle. Balance and coordination improve.

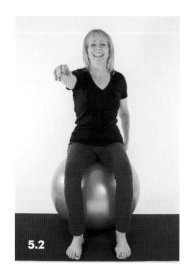

5.2

Bounce in Rhythm 2: Arm Swings

Bouncing to a metronome is a great warm-up exercise and hones your ability to keep a steady tempo. Added arm and leg movements develop balance and coordination, as well, so you can ride with feel at any gait.

1 Set a metronome to about 96 beats per minute.

2 Sit on an exercise ball in upright posture (as you do for *Bounce in Rhythm 1*, p. 21).

3 Bounce to the beat of the metronome.

4 Add a rhythmic, alternating front-and-back swing of your arms (fig. 5.2).

Work for precision: Stay absolutely with the beat. Try to land the same way on the ball each time. For variation, try the next two exercises.

Bounce in Rhythm 3: Toe Tapping

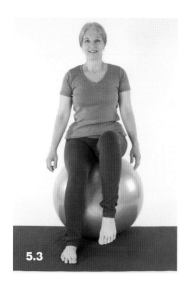

5.3

1 Continue bouncing to the metronome.

2 Keeping your arms still, lift one leg a bit, and tap the foot in rhythm with the metronome (fig. 5.3).

3 Try to keep your balance on the ball using your core muscles so that moving one leg does not disrupt your alignment (like on the horse).

4 Once you gain steady balance tapping one foot, change to tapping the other (you'll probably find it easier to tap one foot compared to the other).

5 When this is straightforward, add tapping one foot for a set number of beats, then switch and tap with the other foot.

6 End by alternating foot taps, like marching.

Bounce in Rhythm 4: Ball Jacks

1 Continue bouncing to the metronome.

2 Swing both arms overhead and back down by your sides, like the arm movements of a jumping jack, for several bounces (fig. 5.4 A).

3 Next, alternate the swinging of your arms (fig. 5.4 B).

4 Then, with quiet arms, move your legs out to the side and back in with the metronome rhythm (fig. 5.4 C). Keep your knees aligned over your feet. Do this several times.

5 When this is stable, alternate your legs: your left leg stays in front of you while your right leg goes out to the side and vice versa (fig. 5.4 D).

6 Finally, combine the arm swings and leg jumps together, like jumping jacks (fig. 5.4 E). For more of a challenge, move your arms alternately (fig. 5.4 F). Then move your legs alternately (fig. 5.4 G). Then move both arms and legs alternately (fig. 5.4 H).

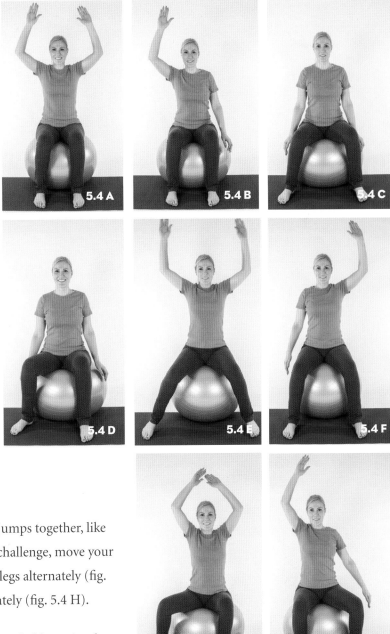

With some of these movements, you will probably notice that it seems like the metronome tempo changes. Isn't it interesting how challenging it is to keep a steady tempo, even in the controlled setting of sitting on a ball? These exercises develop coordination, balance, and your ability to maintain a steady rhythm and perceive subtle deviations from what is desired so you can support your horse in steady gaits.

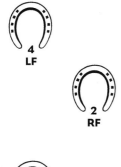

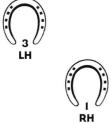

5.5 *The walk's footfall (LH = left hind, RH = right hind, LF = left front, RF = right front).*

Walk

The walk is a four-beat gait. The order of footfall is right hind (RH), right fore (RF), left hind (LH), left fore (LF), as shown in Figure 5.5. There is no moment of suspension at the walk; the horse always has at least two legs on the ground. Therefore, there is no "bounce" or impulsion in the walk, unlike trot and canter.

The alternate stepping of the horse's hind legs causes his whole body to move. As the horse's RH steps under his body, his rib cage swings to the left. As the horse's LH steps under his body, his rib cage swings out of the way to the right. This causes a side-to-side rocking of the horse's rib cage and back, directly under where the rider sits. Watch a horse walk away from you and you'll see this side-to-side rib cage swing (it is particularly obvious in a fat horse or a pregnant mare). Watch a horse from the side and you'll see the back dip down and up as the hind legs step alternately under the body. While the degree of swing in the rib cage varies depending upon scope of the walk and the horse's conformation, it is there, to a certain degree, in all horses.

Learning the rhythm of the walk and how your horse's body moves helps you sit precisely with your horse. When a hind leg steps under the body, you will feel your thighbone on the same side dip slightly down or in, and your opposite thighbone lift up or out slightly. The hip joint on the leg that is lifted up extends open a bit. With practice, you'll feel the alternate hind legs stepping by perceiving the slight rocking of your legs from side to side, and you will start "walking with your horse." When exploring this movement, be careful not to create the movement in your body, but let your horse's body move yours. The movement is not huge, but if you do not allow your legs to swing in this way, in essence, you are telling your horse not to

WALK: What Moves and What Shouldn't Move Much
Your shoulder and elbow joints move to stay with your horse's head and neck.
Your legs alternately swing slightly in and out at the hip joint, staying with your horse's rib cage as it rocks side to side with each step.
Your pelvis and spine move somewhat forward and back (but this is often exaggerated). The amount of movement of your pelvis when you ride a walking horse is similar to the amount of movement of your pelvis when you walk.

RIDER'S CHALLENGE ||||||||||||||||||||||||||||||||||||||||||||||||||||||||||||||||||||||||||||||||||||||||||||||||||||

Working Too Hard at Walk

I arrive at the clinic site and meet Susan who is warming up her seven-year-old Swedish gelding, Jasper. The horse is clearly unfocused in the new environment, but Susan tactfully goes about helping him settle by riding bending lines and transitions. She is clearly a focused and pleasantly empathetic rider. Her posture and balance are reasonably good, but her aids at times cause tension.

"Sometimes I feel Jasper and I are not on the same page. I try to be tactful, but I feel that my aids often disrupt his way of going and communication is a struggle," Susan explains. "Sometimes he tries to listen, and other times I don't have his attention at all."

Remedy

My plan for Susan is to review "what moves and what shouldn't move much" at each gait so she can feel more a part of Jasper's body and apply her aids at a logical time. We start at walk.

I watch Jasper start off walking actively on the track. After a few moments, his energy fades and he looks up and hollows his back. Susan squeezes her legs against his sides to urge him forward. He doesn't answer but continues looking away, remaining quite hollow. She adds more leg squeezing and tucks her pelvis a bit as she tries to get him to walk on, tightening her gluteal muscles and pumping with her butt. Jasper remains hollow and further tightens his back against her aids. His walk gets quick, tense, and pace-like, losing its clear four-beat rhythm.

In this circumstance, the timing and nature of Susan's aids are not effective and disrupt Jasper's way of going. Her leg aids are not rhythmic and are applied against his movement. Her tight and pumping gluteal muscles cause further tension in Jasper's back.

I review with Susan the characteristics of the walk. I lead Jasper (so Susan needn't worry about steering or energy) and Susan feels the swing of her legs with Jasper's rib cage. I encourage her to replace the back-front movement of her pelvis with more side-to-side swinging of her legs at the hip joint. This helps her pelvis remain quiet and helps her feel the walk rhythm. I then give the reins back to her, and she tries to keep the rhythmic movement in her body. When Jasper's walk begins to fade, I coach Susan to give smaller, quicker, and more rhythmic aids from her lower leg only, without using her gluteal muscles much. Further, I guide Susan to use her leg to ask for more energy when Jasper's respective hind leg is stepping under his body and is in the air, not when it is bearing weight: That is, her right leg asks for more walk as Jasper's right hind leg swings under his body, and her left leg asks for more walk as Jasper's left hind leg swings under his body. I also have Susan count the stepping of Jasper's hind legs (1-2-1-2) so she mentally and physically "walks with him" every step.

With Susan's more organized approach to encouraging an active walk, Jasper maintains a rhythmic gait with less tension, and his ears turn backward, listening to her. Susan gives smaller aids to keep an active walk, as she quickly perceives when the walk loses energy. Mentally, she works harder to feel what is happening, but physically she doesn't have to work as hard because her aids are well timed.

Exercises for Susan: *Bounce in Rhythm 1–4; Leg Circles; Leg Lifts on Ball.*

walk. You must support the rhythm and character of the walk to be clear to your horse that this is what you want. Every step.

Feel how the rocking of your horse's rib cage moves your thighbone at your hip joint, rather than at your pelvis. Your pelvis most certainly moves slightly during the walk, both side-to-side as well as front to back and in rotation, but it is easy to exaggerate this pelvic movement and end up moving more than your horse. I encourage some pelvic stability so it stays balanced over your horse's movement.

Now that you feel your legs swinging with your horse's walking steps, you can learn to identify which of your horse's hind legs is stepping under his body. You can check yourself by either looking in a mirror or watching your horse's shoulders (the foreleg on the same side will immediately follow the hind leg). Why learn this skill? Your horse's hind leg is best influenced when it is off the ground and *not* bearing weight. It is off the ground when it steps under his body. By knowing when each hind leg steps under your horse's body, you can improve the timing of your leg aids. It is much more likely that your horse will respond appropriately if you ask for more forward reach or a sideways step when his leg is in the air. Stated another way, if you ask for a sideways step from a hind leg when it is on the ground and bearing weight, your horse cannot respond to the aid and will either tune out or resist. Awareness of the stepping hind legs puts precision in the timing of your aids and is a key element of feel.

Awareness of the rhythm and stepping of your horse's legs also helps you maintain steady activity in the walk. Call out the stepping of your horse's hind legs and keep a steady tempo of these steps marching in your head like a metronome. For simplicity, limit the counting to the hind legs (1-2-1-2) as opposed to all four legs (1-2-3-4-1-2-3-4). With this background rhythm, you will quickly perceive when the horse's energy or tempo changes, and you can give small urging or restraining aids to keep the gait steady. This puts you in a positive and proactive "ride what you want" mindset while you *appear* to be doing very little. This organization is far preferable to large, obvious, and unbalancing corrective aids.

The horse's neck and head undulate at the walk. Again, watch a horse at liberty and you will see how the head and neck move as part of the walk—the horse's mane will swish back and forth. This is the horse's natural gait. You must allow this movement by avoiding stiff and still arms: Your arms must move at the elbow and shoulder joints to keep contact through the bridle elastic and steady. Your horse should not be punished each step by hitting the bit. The amount of your horse's movement, and hence, your arms, will depend upon your horse and the character of his walk. Test yourself to see if you are suitably staying with the movement of your horse at the walk by trying to maintain an even pressure on your fingers from the reins during all steps of the walk.

When it comes to riding the walk, the most common problem I see is the horse training the rider to work too hard! I see this in two ways: First, the rider overuses the gluteal muscles, and second, the rider gives driving leg aids every step of the walk. Both are sort of "wishful thinking" walking that makes you work harder than your horse. Your horse's part of the bargain is to walk; your part of the bargain is to ask the horse for the walk you want and pay close attention to the horse's walk so you can make adjustments should your horse deviate from that.

Trot

The trot is a two-beat gait with a moment of suspension between each beat. The horse's legs move in diagonal pairs: RH with LF, and LH with RF, as shown in Figure 5.6. While the walk carries the horse and rider forward, the trot carries the horse and rider *up*, as well as *forward*—this increased energy at the trot challenges balance in the novice rider.

Just as in the walk, in the trot the horse's hind legs move alternately. As such, there is the same side-to-side swing of the horse's rib cage and back. This will be discussed in more detail when I consider strategies for sitting the trot (see p. 172).

Unlike the walk, at the trot your horse's head-and-neck carriage is quite stable. As such, your hands need to stay relatively still. By this I mean that if you

5.6 *The trot's footfall.*

TROT: What Moves and What Shouldn't Move Much
POSTING TROT
Your hands stay in a stable position.
Your legs stay stable underneath your body.
Your torso is in neutral alignment, slightly inclined forward, while it moves up and forward over the pommel of the saddle, and then back down.
SITTING TROT
Your hands stay in a stable position.
Your legs stay stable underneath your body.
Your torso is in neutral alignment.
Your hip joints allow the side-to-side swing of your legs with your horse's barrel.
Your ankle joints move to absorb the up-and-down motion of the gait.

could put a measuring stick from your hand to your horse's neck or withers, the distance would remain constant during the trot (assuming a reasonably steady head-and-neck carriage on the part of your horse). Your horse's head and neck lack the back-and-forth movement of walk and canter. A common problem in the trot is your arms and hands "posting" up and down or bouncing during the sitting trot. This will antagonize the connection with your horse, and you will be unable to give subtle rein aids. The trot requires you to move your body in the up-and-down motion of the trot while keeping your hands quiet. This happens when your body is balanced and there is suppleness in your shoulder and elbow joint muscles.

EXERCISE for Supple Elbows

The following *Bounce with Dowel* exercise will help you develop the feel for the elbow suppleness needed to keep quiet hands while your body moves with the horse's trot. It is a very subtle feeling, and one I highly recommend be practiced off your horse. He will appreciate your quieter hands!

Bounce with Dowel
Refine your ability to keep your hands steady when you are moving up and down, a skill needed for trot work.

1 Sit on an exercise ball in neutral spine alignment.

2 Hold a 3-foot dowel or stick (a riding crop or whip will do) in your hands out in front of you, elbows bent by your sides (fig. 5.7 A).

3 Start bouncing on the ball. You will see that the dowel bounces up and down with you.

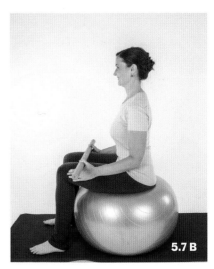

5.7 A

4 Now rest your hands and dowel on your knees. Bounce again (figs. 5.7 B & C). You will notice that since your knees are not going up and down, the dowel's position stays stable, and your elbow joints move as you bounce. This is the feeling you are after when riding either the posting or sitting trot. Your hands stay still while your body goes up and down.

5 Lift your hands off your legs so they are again in the air holding the dowel.

6 Now, as you bounce, try to keep your hands and the dowel still in space (fig. 5.7 D).

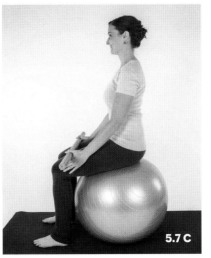

5.7 C

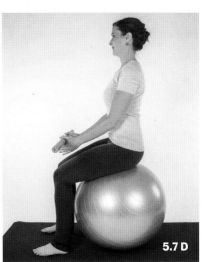

5.7 D

Keeping your hands and the dowel still in space while your body bounces up and down requires awareness and movement at the elbow joints. If this is too hard, have someone hold the dowel still to help you feel the subtle movement at your elbow joints. Alternately tighten your arm muscles so the dowel (and your hands) bounce with you, then release these muscles so the dowel stays still while you bounce; your elbow joints move to allow stillness of your hands and the dowel.

A Pretty Picture

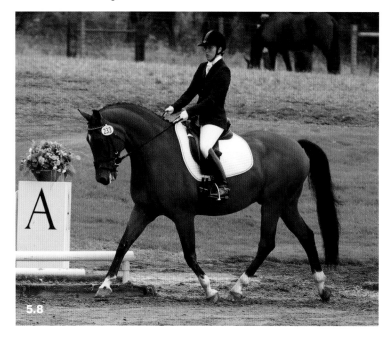

5.8

Jessica Rattner rides "V" in trot keeping correct posture and leg position. You can almost imagine Jessica proactively counting out V's trot steps to keep him reaching underneath his body with his hind legs. This not only keeps his tempo steady, but it also keeps him focused on Jessica. If Jessica backs off from riding every step, V loses focus. Jessica offers a steady hand allowing V to reach for the bit with confidence. Exercises to facilitate this balanced riding include: Abdominal Curls; Spine Extension; Plank on Mat: Knees; Plank on Mat: Feet; Knee Circles; Leg Circles; and Hug-a-Tree: Single Arm.

RIDER'S CHALLENGE ||||||||||||||||||||||||||||||||||||||||||||||||||||||||||||||||||||||||||||||||||||||||||||||||||||

Use Balance for Tempo Control

Leslie comes to my clinic to get another point of view on the challenges involved in riding her ex-park horse Morgan mare, Sprinx, in dressage. I explain that my focus is on her, not her horse training.

"I'm open to any input," she replies.

I watch the two ride some trot circles and see that Leslie finds it difficult to keep Sprinx in a steady trot. Leslie's leg position tends to be too far forward, and her pelvis is too far back in the saddle; she compensates by leaning forward. Sprinx tends to run in the trot, getting quicker and quicker in her tempo until Leslie pulls on the reins, shoving her feet forward, and worsening her imbalance.

The habit that the two of them have now is that Sprinx runs; Leslie pushes into her feet, sending her behind Sprinx's movement; Sprinx loses balance and trots faster; and Leslie pulls on the reins. Sprinx is changing Leslie's balance and body position and until this is fixed, Leslie can't control Sprinx's trot.

Remedy

I have Leslie halt and show her a better leg position and torso alignment. I teach her *Rib Cage Breathing* to keep her focused on maintaining balance from her body's center. I explain how rather than pushing into her feet to steady Sprinx's trot, she can use the movement of her body to stabilize Sprinx's trot, with help from the reins.

Back on the rail, with Leslie's leg positioned underneath her and her body in upright alignment, I have the two of them proceed in a slow posting trot.

Tuning into the stepping of your horse's hind legs is very important at the trot, as horses are often unsteady in their tempo. Feeling and riding a steady metronome-like 1-2-1-2 rhythm from your balanced center (core) facilitates a stable tempo in your horse.

Posting Trot

In posting trot, your torso comes forward over the pommel of the saddle and then rests back down into the saddle in the trot rhythm. It is traditionally taught that you rise out of the saddle when your horse's outside foreleg and inside hind leg are stepping forward and are in the air, and you sit in the saddle when the opposite diagonal pair steps forward. The rise out of the saddle is accomplished by extending both knee and hip joints (angles at the joints *increase*), and flexing them (angles at the joints *decrease*) as you return to the saddle. Neutral spine alignment is maintained during the posting trot.

I coach Leslie to count the trot steps and to try to keep her body moving in a stable tempo.

Leslie successfully counts the steps for about a half circle, then Sprinx speeds up: She loses focus on the tempo, pushes her feet forward, pushes her pelvis back, leans her torso forward, and pulls on the reins.

I point out to Leslie that Sprinx's changing trot changes her. She will not have control of Sprinx's trot until she establishes a much more stable body position.

Leslie is frustrated by Sprinx's behavior, but sticks with it. We go back to counting, and I add my voice so Leslie hears this frame of reference while she struggles to break her habit of becoming unbalanced with Sprinx's unsteady trot tempo. Using the rib cage breathing techniques and counting, Leslie steadies her body position.

Sprinx snorts her annoyance at Leslie's improved presence. While Sprinx struggles to change Leslie, Leslie sticks to her guns to maintain a steady rhythm and position. After a few trot circles, Sprinx begins to come around and trot with a much steadier tempo (slower than her first choice) and better balance.

Leslie demonstrates two important factors necessary for good riding: First, do not let your horse change your position, and second, ride the gait you want, not the varied gait your horse offers. Be clear in your own mind about the gait you want, and put yourself in the rhythm and tempo of that gait. Your horse, with practice, will match you.

Exercises for Leslie: *Bounce in Rhythm 1–4; Pelvic Rocking on Ball: Front to Back; Leg Lifts on Ball; Hug-a-Tree: Both Arms and Single Arm.*

I am riding DG at trot with my leg positioned directly underneath me. This facilitates balance at both posting and sitting trot. I think my posture could be a bit more upright through the upper back, and my neck stretched a bit longer. I know I am tending to lean back because DG can dive downhill in the corners. But, my strategy is not a good one. I need to stay balanced to help her balance. I need to do a few more daily Spine Extension: Scarecrow and Plank on Mat: Feet exercises!

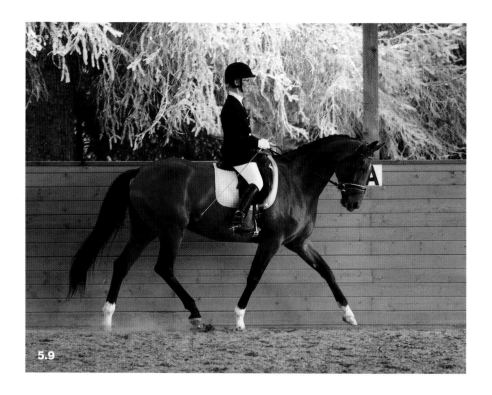

5.9

A correct and stable leg position is important during posting trot. With the shoulder-hip (pelvis)-heel line in place in the down phase, the stirrup acts as a platform for you to step onto in the rising phase. Your leg must stay stable under you to provide a support for the rising phase of the posting trot (fig. 5.9). Without a stable leg position and correct posture, balance is difficult, and you risk falling either behind or ahead of your horse—at worst, using the reins for balance, and at best, ineffectively guiding your horse's trot.

Posting trot has some similarities to the *Pelvic Bridge* exercises (presented in chapter 3). The movement is similar, and the focus of the power for the lift coming through the back of the upper thigh, balanced by the torso, is valuable. However, little power needs to come from you: The horse provides the energy to lift you out of the saddle. But when you precisely direct it through your body, you maintain balance.

A common problem seen at posting trot is an unstable spine position with restricted movement at the hip and knee joints. If hip and knee joint movement is restricted, excessive movement and instability of spine alignment

Unstable Leg Position at Posting Trot

David asks for help with balance on his new horse. Winchester is a 12-year-old, 17.1-hand Hanoverian gelding that has shown through Prix St. Georges. David has ridden much of his life, mostly casual trail riding. In recent years he has been studying dressage, and he purchased this schoolmaster to advance his dressage education.

I watch the two of them warm up. Winchester is a big horse with somewhat lanky gaits, but his temperament is very steady. David rides with a positive and fun attitude, although his lack of attention to detail creates a disorganized picture.

We start working on the posting trot. David adopts a common pattern. As he rises out of the saddle, his feet come forward (his knees straighten). This puts his center of gravity behind his horse's motion, and he falls back heavily in the saddle, sometimes hitting Winchester in the mouth. Winchester responds by slowing his trot and bracing his neck. David kicks Winchester on, but his unstable leg position while posting results in his falling back again, so the cycle continues.

Remedy

At the halt, I hold Winchester's reins and have David rise out of the saddle, as if posting. This is hard to do! Thinking of the *Pelvic Bridge* exercises helps David get the power for the lift from the back of his thigh (hamstring muscles). He first has to hang on to Winchester's mane to rise up out of his stirrups, because he does not keep his feet stable underneath

him. When I stabilize one of his feet in underneath him, David feels how much easier it is to rise out of the saddle. Gradually, I stop supporting his foot and he is able to let go of the mane. To clearly demonstrate what has been happening to him while posting, while David is out of the saddle (still at halt), I move one of his feet forward—and he immediately falls back in the saddle.

Back out on the rail at trot, I have David access the feeling of a stable foot underneath his body, as well as the lift of his body out of the saddle coming through the back of his upper thigh in the hamstring-muscle region. This allows him to stay in better balance, and his center of gravity stays with Winchester's motion. As a result, contact through the bridle is much steadier, and Winchester can trot forward more freely.

As a final challenge to test his stability at posting trot, I have David rise out of the saddle and stay up for one extra beat (essentially changing his posting diagonal by staying out of the saddle for an extra beat rather than sitting an extra beat). First, I have him grab the mane with one hand so any loss of balance is not transmitted to Winchester by pulling on the reins. He finds it remarkably challenging to find the correct balance point at the top of the rise so that he can stay there for a beat. But once he finds it and repeats the exercise without holding on to the mane, his overall balance at posting trot vastly improves, and Winchester's trot settles into a steadier rhythm.

Exercises for David: *Pelvic Bridge* series.

results. When considering "what moves and what shouldn't move much" in the posting trot, the vertebrae of the spine should move very little with respect to each other; the bulk of the movement for posting comes from the hip and knee joints. You know this is happening when the distance between your rib cage and your pelvis stays the same throughout the posting trot cycle. While the spine stays in neutral alignment there is, at posting trot, a slight forward position of the entire torso. But this forward position comes from a change in the angle at the hip joint, not from a change in spine alignment.

Sitting Trot

Sitting the trot is a most challenging skill for a developing rider. It is the gait most likely to trigger detrimental balance strategies, such as gripping with the legs and tightening the shoulders.

RIDER'S CHALLENGE ||||||||||||||||||||||||||||||||||||||||||||||||||||||||||||||||||||||||||||||||||||||||||||

Unstable Spine at Posting Trot

Rebecca, a high school student who is passionate about dressage, spends every extra moment of her busy life at the barn riding her horse—or anyone else's horse that needs some exercise—and helping out with chores. Occasionally, however, she complains to her mother that her back is sore after riding. Her mother contacts me to see if I have any thoughts about what could be causing the strain. Of note, Rebecca is 5 feet, 10 inches tall and weighs about 120 pounds. While many admire her long legs, her long torso is a challenge to support.

I watch Rebecca ride the seven-year-old Thoroughbred gelding, Tipper. Rebecca has a positive approach and, in general, a good sense of where her body should be. As I watch her warming up in posting trot, however, I see how her mechanics are

not doing her spine any favors. Rebecca adopts a pattern of posting that accomplishes the back-and-forth movement of her body during posting by moving at the intervertebral joints of her spine, rather than at the hip and knee joints. As a result, her hip angle, which should open in extension at the top of the rise, moves very little. Instead, at the top of the rise, her abdomen presses forward and her spine extends (arches). Her spine flexes (rounds) when she returns to sitting in the saddle.

Remedy
I explain to Rebecca the importance of maintaining spine alignment and moving at the hip and knee joints to accomplish the posting trot. As with David (see The Rider's Challenge: "Unstable Leg Position

A Pretty Picture

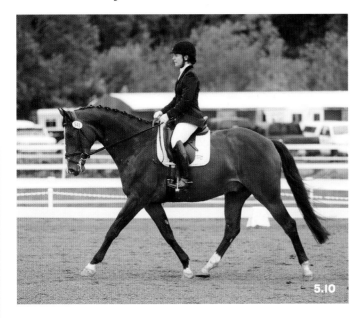

5.10

Paula Helm shows correct spine alignment riding the 2008 Hungarian Warmblood HS Wroyal Prince down the centerline. This young horse benefits from Paula's balance and positive focus. Paula describes Prince as a bit lazy, and she needs to be careful that each of her leg aids has a clear "end" so that her leg releases after sending him forward. With this in mind, I would encourage Paula to move her lower leg very slightly back so it is precisely underneath her—in this photo, her left lower leg is slightly in front of the ideal position. This risks causing her to fall behind Prince, which will not encourage forward movement. All the Pelvic Bridge exercises are great exercises to gain awareness and control of leg position and function.

at Posting Trot," p. 171), I have Rebecca practice the posting trot movement at the halt. It is difficult for her to feel that her spine is doing most of the moving. It is only when I move her pelvis forward over the pommel that she begins to feel that her hip joint can move when she posts out of the saddle. I have Rebecca place her hand on the front of her abdomen to get a sense of the distance between her rib cage and pelvis. She begins to feel that she lets this distance get too long as she posts out of the saddle (arching her spine, see fig. 2.37, p. 58), and then lets this distance get too short as she returns to sitting in the saddle (rounding her spine, see fig. 2.33, p. 54).

Keeping her hand "calipers" on her abdomen for feedback, she begins to keep more stability in her spine alignment and find greater freedom of movement in her hip and knee joints. I guide Rebecca to feel the energy from the horse coming into her body through the back of her upper thigh (hamstring region). Previously, she was feeling and gaining the lift of her body mostly through her low and mid back. This strategy not only is inefficient but could also contribute to her back pain.

Back on the rail, Rebecca practices feeling freedom in her hip angle and a more stable alignment in her spine. All goes well until Tipper gives a little spook, at which point Rebecca's legs grip and she loses the movement at the hip joint. Now, however, she feels the change in her body and goes back to a more supported posture.

Exercises for Rebecca: *Pelvic Bridge: Simple; Plank on Mat: Knees and Feet; Plank on Ball; Quadruped: Single and Diagonal; Leg Circles.*

I have four strategies to help master the sitting trot:

1 First, don't fight the bounce. Don't try *not* to bounce—most everything you'll try will make the bouncing worse. Recognize that the trot has up-and-down movement to it. Rather than not bouncing, think of lifting your body up and forward with the horse. And remember, the bouncing you experience rarely looks as bad as it feels.

2 Second, maintain correct alignment and self-carriage in the trot. Rather than wait for the horse to lift or send you out of the saddle, lift yourself up with the horse. Think "trot with me" to the horse, rather than trying to protect yourself from the movement of the trot. Use the metronome in your head to count the 1-2-1-2 stepping of the horse's hind legs to proactively stay with the horse as opposed to being tossed about by the horse. Emphasizing the *up* phase of the sitting trot promotes this self-carriage and sense of "trotting with the horse." Focusing on staying *down* in the saddle is rarely a successful strategy.

3 Third, use the seat-belt-like tool of the deep abdominal muscles to help anchor your pelvis to the back of the saddle so you go up and down with the saddle: Imagine laces stitching the front of your lower abdomen to the cantle of the saddle as your deep abdominal muscles provide an effective and positive tool to help you stay with your horse at sitting trot. Plus, it is something to tell your body to *do*. So often we are saying *don't*: "Don't tighten the shoulders," "Don't grip with your knees," and so on. But your arms and legs are trying to keep you in the saddle by gripping. Until you replace gripping with an alternate and successful strategy—by focusing on your abdominal "seat belt"—this tension will remain. The abdominal muscle stability organizes the rest of your body so that you can recognize and reduce unnecessary tension. When using this abdominal seat belt, however, avoid changing your spine alignment into a pelvic tuck—stay in neutral spine alignment (fig. 5.11).

4 And fourth, find the side-to-side rhythmic swing of your horse's body to move with it in a positive way. This swing of your horse's barrel, or rib cage, is similar to what happens at the walk. The challenge, however, is that the sitting-trot tempo is much faster than the walk tempo. It takes practice to feel and stay with this rapid motion. As in the walk, I emphasize the movement of your thighbone at the hip joint with this swinging to help keep a stable pelvic and torso position. Again, it is not that the pelvis is immobile, but it is easy for it and the spine to move too much in the sitting trot.

A Pretty Picture

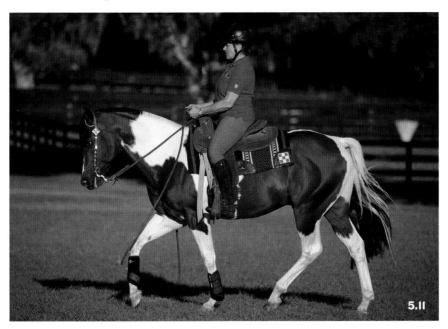

5.11

Lynn Palm shows correct, upright neutral spine alignment in sitting trot while riding Rugged Painted Lark. Lynn describes this horse as "laid back" and says she needs to stay focused, with a "trot-with-me" mindset to keep him stepping actively underneath her. If he waivers from the trot she wants, she is quick to correct with a leg aid so he learns to keep that trot. Lynn's balance and correct posture help make her driving aids clearly understood. Further, her balance prevents her legs from gripping, which would discourage Rugged Painted Lark from trotting forward. You can develop this balance and control at sitting trot with exercises that develop core support (Abdominal Curls; Spine Extension on Mat; Plank on Mat: Knees; Plank on Mat: Feet) and suppleness at the hip joint (Knee or Leg Circles).

As you develop the sitting trot, focus on the first three strategies I describe on p. 174: When your *core stability*, *balance*, and *self-carriage* are secure, then the hip joint swinging generally follows. Feeling this movement at the hip joints is another positive place for your energy and focus—it is another, "Do this," strategy. You will not be able to feel your horse's back swing at sitting trot if your legs are tight and gripping.

In my experience, because of the quick trot tempo, it is much easier to explore your horse's swinging rib cage and move with this swing if you consider just one of your legs at a time. I suggest you start on a circle in either direction and focus on feeling the lift of your thigh on the outside of your horse when his inside leg steps under the body. This movement is more obvious than feeling your inside leg dipping down or in. Just as in the walk, in the sitting trot you can teach yourself to feel when each hind leg steps under your horse's body (see p. 162). Then, your leg aid for either more reach, or a lateral step, can be timed for when your horse's leg is off the ground, and he can answer the aid. Your aids can become more subtle and accurate. Aids not applied in rhythm risk causing tension in your horse. Aids given in rhythm improve the chance that your horse will answer correctly. Thoughtful aids help you work less physically by thinking more instead. Timing your aids correctly develops feel and harmony.

A discussion of sitting trot is not complete without considering the quality of the horse's trot. The better the horse's balance, connection, and engagement, the more the trot movement is taken in the horse's body, and not in the rider's body. There are many considerations, but all things being equal, to protect my back, I avoid sitting the trot on a given horse until he has attained a degree of suppleness and connection so that the trot is not jarring.

Consider "what should move and what shouldn't move much" at sitting trot. The lumbar spine is *not* a place to seek movement in the sitting trot. Doing so risks excess strain and wear and tear on the intervertebral discs and the facet joints. So, do not absorb the movement of the sitting trot in your back.

Stabilize Your Spine for a Pain-Free Sitting Trot

My strategies for sitting the trot have helped riders who've come to me looking for ways to avoid back pain from the trot. Most often I observe instability of the spine in these riders—that is, there is too much motion between the vertebrae of the spine, especially the lower back. Improving spine stability with a strong, engaged set of core muscles often helps reduce back pain from riding.

MY CHALLENGE ||||||||||||||||||||||||||||||||||||||||||||||||||||||||||||||||||||||||||||||||||||

Learning "What Moves and What Shouldn't Move Much" at Walk and Trot

Two horses helped me to clarify my ideas about "what should move and what shouldn't move much" at walk and trot: Mac, a veteran 15.2-hand, Appaloosa gelding, and a similarly mellow Morgan gelding that I leased for my "riding rehab" after I recovered from back surgery.

On Mac, I spent time at walk feeling how his body moved and how I moved with it. I felt his swinging rib cage and struggled to link this movement with his steps. I'd ask myself which hind leg was stepping under his body. I'd speak a rhythm: right-left-right-left. Then I'd check to see if I was correct by looking at his shoulder. If I was incorrect, I'd watch his shoulder or his croup and visually determine when his hind legs were swinging under his body. I'd put in my head the correct "right-left-right-left" stepping and then feel what my body was doing. In this way I could correctly link the movement of my body with his. From this came the images I offer in this book of how to feel when each hind leg steps under your horse's body at walk and trot.

I practiced sitting trot on the Morgan, a more schooled dressage horse. By this time I knew that maintaining proper alignment was absolutely key to limiting further damage to my back. I was determined to figure out how to do this. This horse had a reasonable trot to sit and was reliable enough for me to practice sitting trot with one hand on the reins. I placed my other hand on the front of my body like a pair of calipers, measuring

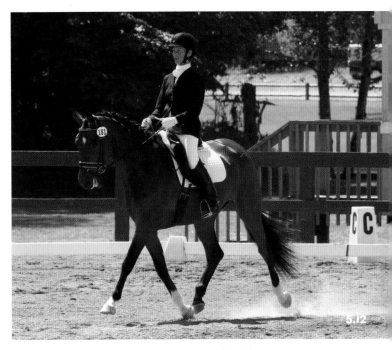

DG and I are doing medium trot in a Second Level test. My "abdominal seat belt" is very useful riding this gait. It would be so easy for me to lean back for stability, but that will only compromise DG's balance. I keep a mantra in my head of "up and forward, up and forward" during the medium trot to try and keep my center of balance over hers. Again, what is my favorite exercise for developing this solid position? Plank on Mat: Knees or Plank on Mat: Feet, of course!

the distance between my ribs and pelvis, and figured out how to keep this distance stable—hence, my spine stable—during sitting trot. With practice came the seat-belt tool (p. 174), as well as awareness of the swing of the horse's rib cage, and my legs at the hip joints (fig. 5.12).

Here I am on DG at sitting trot keeping spine stability and self-carriage with my "abdominal seat belt," and allowing my legs to swing with her back. It is not possible in a still photo to see the swing at my hip joint with her trot, but with each step I check that my thigh moves with her swinging rib cage. Leg Circles is a great exercise to develop suitable suppleness in the hip-joint muscles to feel this movement.

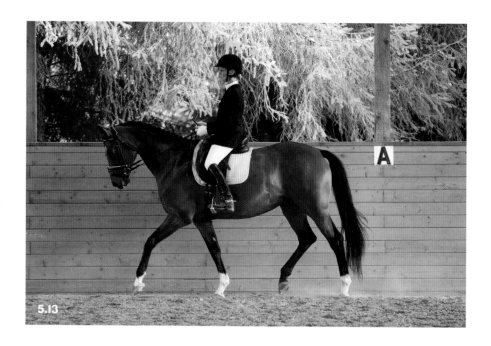

5.13

RIDER'S CHALLENGE

Unstable Spine at Sitting Trot

Remember Rebecca? (See The Rider's Challenge: "Unstable Spine at Posting Trot," p. 172.) This enthusiastic high school student had some challenges maintaining stability of her long torso at the posting trot. Now we move on to the sitting trot.

I am not surprised to see Rebecca's spine move too much at sitting trot. Her tight leg and hip joints lock against Tipper's body, forcing movement into her spine. This gripping also puts her slightly out of sync with Tipper's rhythm; her "up and down" lags Tipper's "up and down."

Remedy

I describe my four strategies for sitting the trot, emphasizing her self-carriage and abdominal seat-belt support. I don't spend a lot of time telling Rebecca to not grip. To me it doesn't make sense to

tell a muscle to release and "let go" when it has taken on the job of keeping you "safe" and stable in the saddle. Rather, I think of the muscles that should be working to keep you in the saddle (your core) and focus on them "doing more." Relaxing the gripping legs without finding a different strategy to stay in the saddle only guarantees the gripping will quickly return.

Back on the rail, I have Rebecca think of lifting herself up out of the saddle with Tipper and carrying herself forward with him. This improves her ability to stay in sync with his trot. I also have her call out loud the 1-2-1-2 stepping of the hind legs. She finds this remarkably hard to do; her rhythm often falls behind Tipper's. But once she gets a more proactive approach to staying with Tipper at the trot, her spine stability improves.

This risks too much movement in the spine in an unhealthy way. A bit of pelvic lift in the *up* phase of the sitting trot is a good strategy, but avoid spine extension (arching) when your weight returns down onto your horse's back as this risks strain.

Again, it is too simple to say that your lumbar spine and pelvis do not move in sitting trot. Most certainly they do. There must be *some* movement in these joints. But, do not absorb the movement of the trot only in these joints. Rather, support the spine and pelvis as much as possible so the *down* forces of the sitting trot do not result in shear strain across the joints of your spine.

Seeking balance and self-carriage, going up and forward in space with your horse, stabilizing your spine with your abdominal seat belt, and finding movement at your hip joints—joints meant to move—are more logical strategies (fig. 5.13). You can check if your spine alignment is stable at sitting

||||||||||||||||||||||||||||||||||||||||||||||||||||||||||||||||||||||||||||||||||||||||||||||||||||||||||||||||||||||||||||||||||||||||||||||||||||||||

Rebecca also needs a lot of help from her abdominal seat belt to support her spine. We review this tool and I encourage her to experiment with how much effort she needs for a more stable body. We again use her hand like a set of calipers on the front of her abdomen so she can feel if her rib-cage-to-pelvis distance changes much with each trot step.

Like many riders, Rebecca discovers that it is easier to feel the positive effect of her abdominal seat belt if her torso is tipped slightly behind the vertical. This helps her feel the horse move out in front of her stable body position. Ideally, in the end, her body will be closer to the vertical, but for now this helps her support her spine. We also start at a relatively slow trot.

After a few rounds of focusing on counting the trot steps and keeping her abdominal seat belt on, her gripping legs begin to release, allowing her thighbones to move with Tipper's barrel. I ask if she can feel this movement.

"Sort of," she answers. "They definitely feel looser than before."

I have Rebecca pick up a circle to the right and settle into a steady rhythm. I coach her to feel her left (outside) thigh lift up as I call out "now" when Tipper's right (inside) hind leg steps forward under his body. From her core stability, and the cue "now" in rhythm with the trot, she can feel how her legs move with Tipper's body. Gradually, Tipper's trot becomes freer and covers more ground as Rebecca's gripping legs release and allow Tipper's back to swing. And, Rebecca enjoys improved spine stability and hip-joint muscle suppleness. Now she is moving with Tipper—and smiling.

Exercises for Rebecca: *Bounce in Rhythm 1–4; Abdominal Curls; Plank on Mat: Knees and Feet; Plank on Ball; Quadruped: Single and Diagonal; Knee Circles; Leg Circles; Leg Lifts on Ball.*

trot by observing or feeling the rib-cage-to-pelvis distance at the front of your body. If this distance is steady, so is your spine alignment.

The challenge of sitting the trot often leads to shoulder tension, precluding suppleness in muscles of the shoulders and elbows. As a result, rather than a quiet hand position, your hands bounce up and down with the trot's movement. At the sitting trot, you must feel as if your arms become part of the bridle and your hands stay steady to your horse's mouth. This is tricky to feel. The movement at the shoulder and elbow that allows a stable hand position at both posting and sitting trot is very subtle. To clarify this skill, I teach a rider to anchor her hands either by pressing her baby finger against either side of the horse's withers or looping her baby finger under a bucking strap. With her hand position stabilized, the rider can then feel the movement necessary at the elbow during posting and sitting trot to accomplish steady contact with the horse. The *Bounce with Dowel* exercise develops this skill off the horse (see p. 166).

RIDING EXERCISE to Improve Sitting Trot

Here is a riding exercise to help you improve your connection with your horse at sitting trot and explore how paying attention to your body facilitates your horse's movement.

1 Establish a circle right at sitting trot. The size can depend upon your level of training, but 15 to 20 meters works well.

2 Establish the tempo of your horse's trot in your head by counting the stepping of his hind legs: 1-2-1-2.

3 Change the 1 and 2 to right and left, matching the hind leg that is stepping under your horse's body. Try to identify which hind leg steps under the body by feeling how your thighbones move at the hip joint. Recall that your outside thighbone will lift up as your horse's inside hind leg steps under his

body. If you aren't sure of the stepping of your horse's hind legs, simply watch his shoulders. Like learning your posting diagonals, the opposite shoulder will come forward with the hind leg in question.

4 Add an emphasis of the stepping under of the inside (in this case, the right) hind leg: *right*-left-*right*-left-*right*-left, and so on. Feel how your body moves with this rhythm. Feel that both your inside (right) thigh dips down, and your outside (left) thigh lifts up when you say "right." This helps your inside leg support your horse's engaging inside-right hind leg, and it helps your outside thigh allow the outward swing of the rib cage. Both help your horse maintain bend and rhythm.

5 Practice this exercise in both directions, emphasizing the inside (*left*) hind leg when tracking left.

6 Finally, establish a figure-of-eight movement with two equally sized circles of 15 to 20 meters. Find the rhythm as described above. Now you will have to change the emphasis of your right-left metronome as you change direction. This is challenging.

As you change direction in the figure-of-eight, switch from *right*-left-*right*-left to *left*-right-*left*-right—again, the emphasis is on the inside hind leg as it reaches under your horse's body. It may take a few steps for you to make the change in emphasis. With practice, you can do it quickly, and develop the skill to support the bend and rhythm of your horse's trot in any direction or change of direction. This skill translates into riding the hind legs appropriately in lateral work.

Unsteady Hands at Trot

Tamara is a petite novice rider well matched to her 15-hand, Arab gelding, Jake. Like many adult riders, she started riding as a kid, and then stopped for school, career, and family. She is motivated to improve her riding as much as possible within her restricted riding schedule.

Tamara and Jake are warming up when I arrive. I watch for a few minutes as they do some walk and trot work. Jake is a willing worker but can be fussy in the contact. Tamara has decent balance but does not always have control of her arms and, at times, conveys a disorganized picture. I note particularly that Tamara's arms move a lot during the posting trot. This is where we start.

Tamara and Jake proceed at walk, and I help Tamara feel Jake's rhythm, rib-cage swing, and particularly, how his head and neck move at the walk. At trot, the energy from Jake's body causes Tamara's shoulders to tighten. As a result, her arm locks and her whole shoulder and arm post up and down with her. Rather than having a stable contact with Jake through the bridle, her hands are moving.

Remedy

I have Tamara reach both of her baby fingers down to Jake's withers so they have a reference point. Then, as Tamara moves off in posting trot, by keeping her hands contacting Jake's body, she begins to feel what it is like for her body, but not her hands, to move up and down in the posting trot. This requires shoulder and elbow suppleness not initially possible because of tension.

We practice several rounds of posting trot in both directions. At times, Tamara succeeds in stabilizing her hands by moving her elbow joints. I give Tamara two images: One is to feel her body swing through her arms; the other is to imagine a tray resting on her forearms. These images help her focus on her body movement and arm stability.

As expected, the sitting trot presents the same problem. Tamara tries not to bounce, and her shoulders tense up around her ears. Her hands bounce with her body with the expected annoyance from Jake, who hollows and moves forward reluctantly.

I review sitting trot strategies with Tamara, emphasizing the abdominal seat belt for security. After a few circles of alternating sitting and posting trot, she isn't quite as stiff, but her hands are still unstable. I again have her rest her hands on Jake's neck for stability and clarity of position. She keeps her hands stable for just a few steps of sitting trot before her shoulder tension returns, pulling Tamara's hands away from Jake's neck.

I advise Tamara to practice a stable hand position at posting trot before working at sitting trot. She begins by doing just a few steps of sitting trot at a time, either by alternating between posting and sitting, or coming to walk. Over time, with improved core stability and awareness, she achieves more control of her arms and hands.

Exercises for Tamara: *Plank on Ball; Plank on Mat: Knees and Feet; Leg Lifts on Ball; Hug-a-Tree: Both Arms and Single Arm; Bounce with Dowel.*

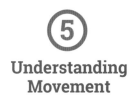

Canter

The canter is a three-beat gait with a moment of suspension, as shown in Figure 5.14. For the right lead, the order of footfall is: LH, RH and LF together, RF, moment of suspension. Unlike the walk and trot in which the hind legs move in opposition to each other, in the canter, the hind legs initially move almost together during the first two beats of the gait. This results in an undulating, rolling path of energy through the horse's back, from the outside hind leg to the inside foreleg.

To find the canter rhythm, focus on the swinging of the hind legs under your horse's body. Think of it as one large beat and say in your head "*can*-ter, *can*-ter, *can*-ter," with the emphasis on the two hind legs swinging under. This emphasis informs the timing of the driving aids: When needed, they should occur on the first beat (*can*) when the hind legs are swinging under your horse's body and can respond.

I have found the canter to be the most variable gait among horses. As discussed, your arms must allow your horse's head and neck to move. And, although your legs should be stable, they can only be still if you have enough suppleness in your hip-joint muscles to allow the undulation of your horse's body to move through this joint. Think of your balanced torso riding the canter much like a bobbing cork or float riding the upward energy of a wave: The float stays on top of the wave and is not disturbed, from a balance standpoint, by the wave. In the same way, you should feel upright on your horse. The nature of your horse's movement at canter encourages your body to move front to back. It is easy for the horse's movement to send your body forward too much—as your horse's hind legs step under and his forehand comes up—and then send your body backward too much—behind the vertical—when he comes down on his leading foreleg. Some of this motion is appropriate, but it should not be exaggerated.

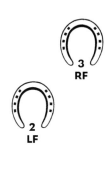

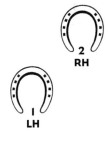

5.14 *The canter's footfall.*

CANTER: What Moves and What Shouldn't Move Much
Your arms follow the motion of your horse's head and neck.
Your legs are stable.
Your hip joints allow the rolling back-to-front motion of your horse's body, especially your inside hip joint.
Your torso stays in correct alignment, without excess rocking forward and back. The more collected the canter, the less your torso rocks; it adopts a more up-and-down motion with your horse.

I am riding DG at left lead canter. While my leg position is okay, I am close to pitching my body too far forward at this phase of the canter. During canter, I call out the rhythm of the gait in my head: "can-ter, can-ter, can-ter." Then, I change the words to: "under-up, under-up, under-up," which helps me encourage her to swing her haunches underneath her body in the first beat of the canter rhythm ("can" or "under") and then encourage her to stay uphill when landing on her leading foreleg on the second beat ("ter" or "up"). Bounce in Rhythm exercises help me keep precise in supporting this steady rhythm in DG's canter.

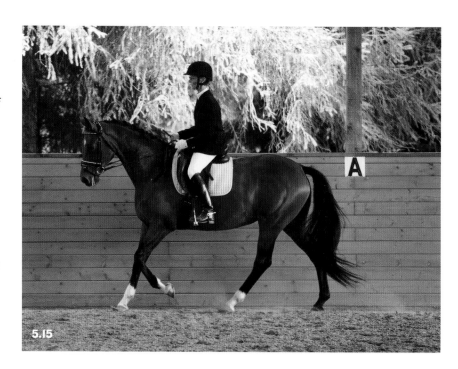

5.15

RIDER'S CHALLENGE ||||||||||||||||||||||||||||||||||||||||||||||||||||||||||||||||||||||||||||||||||||||||||||||||||||||||||||

Stiff Arms and Legs at Canter

Kim is a studious intermediate rider who is always looking for ways to improve her riding. "I feel I need to work hard to keep him going, especially in the canter," she tells me.

I watch Kim ride her eight-year-old, Second-Level, Swedish Warmblood gelding, Oswald. Overall, she has a positive focus, and a fairly correct and strong posture. Her arm and leg positions look a bit forced, as if she works to keep them in place. When I see this, I always go back and reevaluate posture.

I get some ideas for improving Kim's riding efficiency (helping her *think* more and *work* less) at canter. To my eye her arms are quite still, while her upper back, hinging at her waist, presses back in an exaggerated motion as Oswald canters onto his leading foreleg. At the same time, by necessity, there is more arch in Kim's lumbar spine. Kim's hip angle remains fixed.

Kim demonstrates a common scenario at canter: Her hip and shoulder-joint muscles lack suppleness. This is manifest by an exaggerated torso rocking, which causes spine-alignment changes.

Remedy

Three things need to happen to improve Kim's function at canter. First, her arms must allow movement of the horse's head and neck. At halt, I have Kim move her arms forward and back, in line with the bit, to help her appreciate the range of motion the arms can have, and the movement possible at the elbow and shoulder joints. Second, her hip joint must supple and movable so that the

Also, any torso movement should preserve neutral spine alignment; the movement should happen at the hip joints, not at the intervertebral joints (fig. 5.15).

Lateral balance can become quite problematic at the canter. When cantering in a circle, it is challenging to sit in the middle of your horse when the side you tend to sit heavily is on the outside of the circle. It is as if centrifugal force from the canter throws you to the outside. Unfortunately, this unbalances your horse and makes clear aids difficult. In fact, I have observed reluctance from some horses to pick up the correct, inside lead when the rider sits to the outside. Practice establishing lateral balance and symmetry at walk and trot before expecting great things at the canter. And remember, just because it feels odd does *not* mean that it is wrong. Let your horse be your guide and check your position. If your horse tends to fall on his outside shoulder at canter in one direction, check that you are not falling to the outside of the saddle on that side, contributing to the imbalance.

---

canter movement can pass through the joint without disturbing posture. This, of course, can only happen with a more secure understanding of correct posture, which leads to the third challenge: correct postural support. Kim's upper back and body need to stay balanced over her pelvis. For this I explain the same planes image that I used for Jennifer (see The Rider's Challenge: "S-Shaped Posture," p. 64). That is, imagine the upper back in the area of the shoulder blades as one plane, and the abdominal wall as another plane. The upper-back plane needs to press forward at the same time the abdominal-wall plane presses back. These actions decrease the excess upper-back flexing (rounding) and lumbar-spine extending (arching) Kim adopts during the canter.

Kim bravely experiments first with moving her arms more and letting her legs rest on the stirrups with less gripping. At first, she exaggerates her arm movement, which I think is a good thing. She hones in on an amount of movement that allows a steady contact with Oswald. With improved arm suppleness, she improves her posture by bringing both her upper back plane and her lower abdominal plane toward the middle of her body. Improved posture allows improved movement in her hip joints. Amazingly, Oswald bounds more freely upward and forward in the canter. Horses are so sensitive! A seemingly small change in how Kim organizes her body makes a world of difference in his way of going.

Exercises for Kim: *Plank on Ball; Plank on Mat: Knees and Feet; Knee Circles; Leg Circles; Partner Arm Suppleness.*

A Pretty Picture

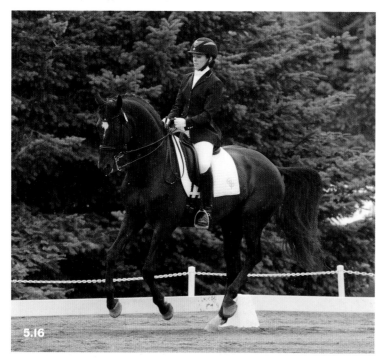

5.16

Catherine Reid demonstrates correct posture and suitable suppleness at the shoulder and hip joints to stay with Skywalker HW's canter. Her elegant position makes it look as if she isn't doing anying—but that is not the case! Catherine describes Skywalker as a bit lazy, but says she needs to be careful and subtle with her aids to keep him active, otherwise he becomes tense. Here, Catherine effectively adapts to Skywalker's movement step by step and makes small adjustments in his balance and energy as needed. The end result looks free and easy, but takes all of the five Rider Fundamentals to accomplish: Mental Focus, Proper Posture, Body Control—Legs and Arms, and Understanding Movement.

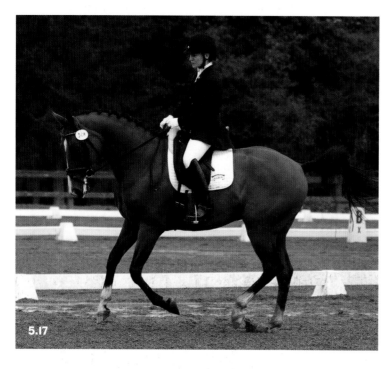

5.17

Paula Helm rides H.S. Whrapsody in canter. Her lack of gripping allows Whrapsody to canter freely forward. Paula explains that the "jump" in Whrapsody's canter improved dramatically as she developed improved control of her legs. She, like many riders, had developed a tendency to "pump" with her gluteal muscles in the canter. Whrapsody responded with back tension and quickly taught her to release her gluteal muscles and use her lower legs to keep his canter active. Helpful exercises for developing this awareness include the Pelvic Bridge exercise series; Knee Circles; and Leg Circles.

RIDER'S CHALLENGE ||||||||||||||||||||||||||||||||||||||||||||||||||||||||||||||||||||||||||||||||||||||||||||||||||||||||

Pumping Gluteal Muscles at Canter

Sheila is a novice adult rider proud to have mastered walk and trot on her 10-year-old Fjord mare, Jade. She now wants to improve their canter.

I watch Sheila and Jade work first at walk and trot. Sheila tends to push with her gluteal muscles at both walk and trot, so when she tries a canter depart with Jade, she uses the same strategy, pumping the pelvis into a tuck with her "glutes," to keep Jade going. The problem is, however, the harder she pumps, the more Jade hollows, breaking from the canter into a fast and bouncy trot.

Remedy

I explain to Sheila that her overworking gluteal muscles are working against her. I start by showing Sheila how much she is using her gluteal muscles at walk and trot. I show her how to focus on using just her lower leg for a driving aid and less of her gluteal muscles (just as I did for Linda and Wendberg; see The Rider's Challenge: "Overusing Gluteal Muscles," p. 100). This requires Sheila to maintain her position in the saddle without gripping legs or tight gluteal muscles. To help her gain awareness of her gluteal muscles tightening, at halt, I have her squeeze them tightly, and then release them.

Back in the canter, I coach Sheila to again use her lower leg as an aid. She struggles with this, as her legs tend to cling to Jade's side in the canter. Without her legs free to give a "go" aid, she is left using her pelvis to try and keep the canter, which is not successful, and Jade falls into a trot.

I coach Sheila in a sitting trot to help her feel her abdominal seat belt stabilize her pelvis to the back of the saddle and to help her feel more secure in her position and balance. This allows her gripping legs to let go. We then go back into canter, and I encourage her to feel her pelvis stay relatively still in the saddle while her legs remain free to aid Jade. We review leg-aid timing: Her legs encourage Jade to canter as the hind legs sweep under Jade's body. I coach Sheila to add a rhythmic tap with her whip when Jade doesn't answer her leg aid. This prevents Sheila from pumping and gripping if Jade doesn't respond to just the lower leg. I have her feel herself going up and forward with Jade in the canter.

These images and tools help Sheila avoid gripping and pumping with her gluteal muscles, and as a result, Jade canters more easily. She quickly is on a positive feedback loop of less pumping, more canter, even less pumping and looser legs, rhythmic leg aids, and a canter that is much easier to maintain.

Exercises for Sheila: *Pelvic Bridge: Simple and Single Leg; Knee Circles; Leg Circles; Leg Lifts on Ball.*

Transitions

Transitions are immensely beneficial for developing balance and self-carriage in your horse and are a fundamental check of your horse's training progress. But remember: You are a part of that team. What can you do to enable your horse to do a balanced transition and not create problems?

There are two components of a transition to consider: *rhythm* and *energy*. A transition may involve a change in rhythm and/or a change in energy. For example, riding a transition from a working trot to a trot lengthening does not involve a rhythm change, but it does involve a change (an increase) in energy. Riding a trot-to-walk transition involves a change in rhythm (trot rhythm to walk rhythm) and a change (decrease) in energy.

Some transitions are tricky, and we could quibble about how to characterize them. For example, is there a change in rhythm or energy going from collected trot to medium trot? The rhythm stays the same. I say there is a change in energy, but the change is more in how the horse *uses* the energy. For collection, the energy is sent more upward, and for the medium trot, it is sent both up and out.

The canter-to-trot transition is also interesting. It is a difficult transition with a clear change in rhythm. I would argue, however, that usually there isn't much of a change in energy—the horse doesn't really slow down going from canter to trot. In fact, slowing the horse down to get from canter to trot impairs the subsequent trot quality.

Regardless of which transition components are most important, you must be ready for the change in your body—in energy and rhythm—and prepare to move appropriately with your horse. This takes focus, postural support, and body control. With organization, you will maximize the benefit of transitions on your horse's balance and make them look effortless and harmonious.

Upward Transitions

In all transitions, you must stay balanced—despite the change in your horse's energy—and move appropriately with the ensuing gait. In *up* transitions, the energy increases. To ride a balanced up transition, anticipate the increased forward energy and avoid being left behind. Establish a proactive mindset, self-carriage from core balance, and a "come with me" intent to encourage the increased energy from your horse. Your leg aids provide the final cues for the up transitions; be ready to move in the rhythm of the new gait.

Downward Transitions

Just as in the up transitions, maintaining balance is key for a good quality *down* transition. Without preparation, a down transition can cause you to fall forward. Most downward transitions result in less forward energy. Use your core muscles to prepare your body for that decreased energy. I think of the front of the body functioning like a wall that tells the horse, "I'm not going forward so much anymore, and neither should you." Basing the down transitions with the intent of your body, supported by your core muscles, assists your balance and prevents an abrupt restricting rein aid. As in the up transition, be prepared to move in the rhythm of the new gait.

A common error in riding down transitions is positioning your body behind the vertical and leaning back, using body weight at times against the reins to facilitate the transition. While appropriate in a bolting runaway horse, it is not appropriate in horse training. Leaning back does not encourage your horse to step underneath you from behind, raise his back, or gain better balance off his forehand. Rather, leaning back encourages your horse to fall on his forehand. In a halt or down transition, if your horse is strong in the bridle, seek strong stability from your torso against the pulling rein and use carefully timed driving aids (legs and intent) to guide the horse to step under himself in better self-carriage. Bending lines and lateral steps help guide the horse to better balance.

Horse training aside, however, it's important that you not let your horse's poor balance change *you*. If you do, you've given your horse the green light to do it again—your horse changed your posture and balance, hence his strategy has been reinforced. You remain effective only when you keep a stable body position despite your horse's actions, reactions, and balance challenges.

Specific Transitions

Walk-to-Halt or Trot-to-Halt Transition

Consider what happens when going from either walk or trot to a halt. You go from moving with your horse as appropriate for the given gait to not moving at all. That is the basis of your halt aid. Stop moving. Breathe to facilitate this transition. For walk to halt, note that your arms and legs are moving with your horse, and your pelvis moves somewhat too. Take an inhale breath, and as you exhale, firm up your core muscles to stabilize your pelvis and anchor your arms by your sides. You needn't pull back to accomplish this transition: simply stop your movement (figs. 5.18 A & B).

The same strategy will work for trot to halt. Your horse will quickly learn this aid. Done this way, the halt aid happens without pulling and promotes

In A, Gail Magnuson stages an unbalanced halt on her 2008 Trakehner mare Luthien (aka "Lula"). Gail incorrectly leans back, tenses her shoulders, and pushes into her feet shoving them forward. These strategies cause Lula to halt on her forehand with a braced neck.

In B, Gail rides a more balanced halt keeping her shoulders aligned over her pelvis, and her feet underneath her. She uses her pelvis as her base of support for the halt rather than her feet. Lula comes to a more balanced halt.

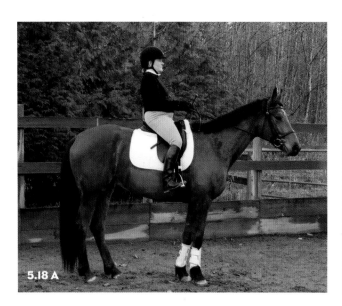

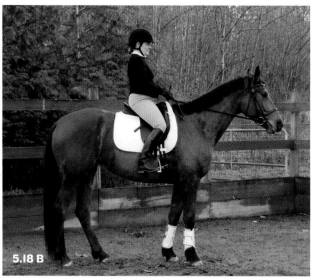

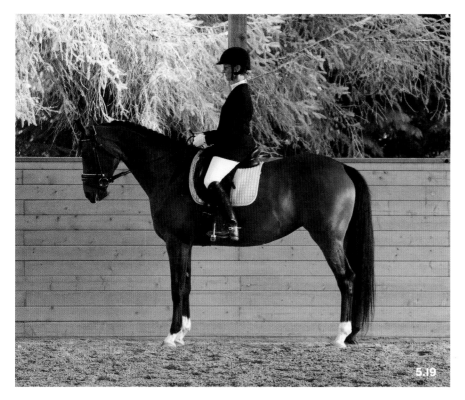

5.19

I stay upright in correct alignment and body position to support DG in a balanced halt from walk. To accomplish this transition, I use an exhale breath (as demonstrated in Rib Cage Breathing 1 and 2) to engage my core muscles and stop my pelvis from moving with DG's back. My rein aid is simply a cessation of staying with her undulating neck at walk. She "hears" these changes and responds with a balanced halt. Use of an exhale breath as the foundation of every restraining aid (as if your body says, "I'm not going forward anymore") allows precision and tact in your restraining rein aids. Useful exercises to develop this coordination include: Rib Cage Breathing 1 and 2; Partner Arm Suppleness; and Partner Arm Stability.

balance and harmony. You appear as if you've done "nothing." But in fact, you've ridden the transition in a thoughtful, organized, balanced, and logical manner. This makes it look easy (fig. 5.19).

Trot-to-Walk Transition

Focus on the change of rhythm that happens when going from trot to walk. As you do with other transitions, use your breath to organize and center, and then add a bit more tone to give that "don't go forward so much" message to your horse. Be prepared to soften your aid as soon as your horse walks so you do not lose energy. Often this transition results in a loss of forward energy— your horse abruptly props himself on his forelegs and then needs to reorganize into the walk.

Try this exercise to improve your trot-to-walk transition.

1 Establish an active trot, either posting or sitting.

2 Initiate the transition to walk not by pulling on the reins, but by slowing how your body moves with your horse—slow your posting or sitting rhythm. Use rib cage breathing to activate your core muscles and balance, and encourage stability and integrity of your body so your horse can hear your change in tempo.

3 Gradually slow your tempo until your horse comes to a walk. You should find that in the resulting walk, your horse moves forward freely.

It may take many trot steps to accomplish the walk transition at first. But, over time, your horse will learn the "don't go forward so much" cue from your body stability and breathing, and quickly come to a prompt, balanced, and active walk. The transition comes from managing your horse's energy from your center and steadying—not pulling on—the reins. This promotes balance and harmony between you and your horse.

Canter-to-Trot Transition

This is a very challenging transition to do well. For this transition, think of going from canter to trot as just a change in rhythm, with little or no change in energy. I use rib cage breathing to prepare (again, your half-halt and the horse's half-halt). Give a short steadying squeeze with the outside rein, exhale, and stabilize your body into an imagined trot rhythm. Sometimes, it takes several tries for your horse to understand the aids for this transition, but basing this transition in your center and focusing on the rhythm change has a beneficial balancing effect on your horse. It makes clear to both you and your horse what is changing. Simply pulling on the reins can result in slowing the canter and losing impulsion, causing your horse to fall into an unbalanced trot.

Canter-to-Walk Transition

This transition requires more skill in terms of timing. It makes most sense to ask for this transition when your horse's hind legs swing under his body so he has a chance to balance on his haunches during the decline in forward motion. Prepare by feeling the canter rhythm. Earlier, I described simplifying the canter rhythm to a two-beat count: *can*-ter, *can*-ter, with *can* being the time when your horse's hind legs swing under, and the *ter* part being when his forehand comes onto the leading foreleg. The aid for the canter-walk transition should come with the *can* to facilitate your horse coming to walk sitting on his haunches. Ride the canter rhythm and use a stabilizing exhale breath to say "don't go forward so much," and anchor your arms by your sides. Soften the rein aid when your horse walks.

Within-Gait Transitions—Up and Down

Within-gait transitions come from maintaining a steady tempo and rhythm (by understanding the horse's gait and using your mental metronome) and modulating the amount of forward versus upward energy. Your body directs the energy *up* for collection, *up and out* for medium gaits, and *out* for extended gaits. Imagine arrows in the middle of your body, one is directed upward (collection) and one is directed outward (extension). Within-gait transitions emphasize one of these arrows in your body (fig. 5.20).

To do a *down* transition from medium trot to collected trot, for example, sit tall and use an exhale breath (this gives both you and your horse a half-halt) to draw your core muscles inward and tell your horse not to go forward so much. At the same time, close your fingers on the reins, but avoid being so strong in the bridle that your horse loses impulsion. Keep a pronounced rhythm in your body and your hip joints, swinging in rhythm to keep your horse in trot, but one that doesn't cover so much ground. Be prepared to give a leg aid or a tap with the whip to encourage your horse to step under into collected trot. For

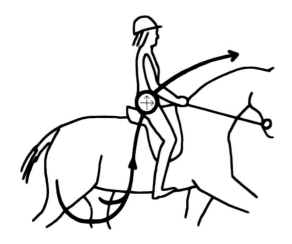

5.20 *This rider-energy diagram shows how the rider, through her center, can direct the horse in varied degrees of upward and forward.*

sure, you may find the need to give a driving aid in the down transition from medium to collected trot so your horse does not lose activity.

To do an *up* transition from collected trot to medium trot, with your horse actively engaged and with you, send energy out in front of you with intent. Support a stable rhythm with your body to counteract your horse's tendency to trot with a quicker tempo rather than with longer, engaged steps. Provide enough stability through the bridle to prevent your horse from falling on his forehand. If your horse needs more forward energy to accomplish the longer trot steps, apply your driving leg aids in rhythm, stay balanced over the center of your horse, and if needed, add a tapping of the whip in rhythm with the gait.

Many riders fall behind the vertical in trot lengthenings, and medium or extended trot. This is not an efficient position, however, because leaning back

RIDER'S CHALLENGE ||||||||||||||||||||||||||||||||||||||||||||||||||||||||||||||||||||||||||||||||||||||||||||||||||||||||||||||||

Balance During Transitions

We earlier met Leslie and Sprinx (see The Rider's Challenge: "Use Balance for Tempo Control," p. 168), who struggle with balance and steadiness at the trot, and with balance in down transitions.

As Leslie and Sprinx work on gaining harmony and a steady trot, I notice that whenever Leslie comes to a walk or halt, balance is a real problem. When I cue her for a down transition, Leslie pushes her feet in front of her and leans back against the reins. The resulting transition is abrupt and on the forehand, with Sprinx propping against her front legs. I wait to work on transitions until Leslie understands the power she has over Sprinx by riding from her center, rather than riding from her feet and hands.

Remedy

I first have Leslie try walk-to-halt transitions using her breath to stabilize her body and prevent a change in her body position—that is, keeping her feet underneath her and not leaning back.

Leslie is skeptical, but gives it a try. On the first few attempts Sprinx wanders a bit. Leslie struggles to not buy into Sprinx's wandering by leaning back and pulling. After three or four tries, however, Leslie feels how simplifying her transition aids from "moving with Sprinx" to "not moving with Sprinx" results in a better balanced and less abrupt halt. Sprinx begins to focus more on Leslie, cocking her ears back in anticipation of the next cue.

encourages your horse onto his forehand. As well, this imperfect alignment requires you to compensate, either through gripping legs or through a restraining rein. Better control comes from correct posture and spine alignment balanced over your horse, moving forward with your horse.

Lateral Movements

The Rider Fundamentals are put to full use tackling the lateral movements—for example, leg-yield, shoulder-in, travers, and half-pass. Focus on the movement at hand, and be sure you know what you are asking for from your horse! Keep precise balance so you can guide your horse sideways. Control the arm and leg aids so they do not put you off balance. Finally, appropriately time your aids with the rhythm of your horse. It is beyond the scope of this book to discuss the details of every lateral movement; I have some general thoughts and will use the leg-yield as an example in the pages that follow.

Adjusting Leslie's strategies for riding trot-to-walk transitions is more challenging. Back in posting trot, I again guide Leslie to good spine alignment with her feet underneath her. I have her ride a walk transition by slowing her posting until Sprinx walks.

I clarify to Leslie that in the end, I am not after a trot-to-walk transition that takes many slowing trot steps, but Leslie can feel that when she rides the transition to walk by slowing the trot, Sprinx does not lose balance and forward direction in the resulting walk. Leslie is forced to keep her balance because she is posting, and Sprinx is forced to keep her balance because Leslie does not offer a rein for her to lean on. The walk that results is forward and active.

I assure Leslie that with practice she will not have to take so much time to get from trot to walk. But done this way, she learns to use her center as the basis of the trot-to-walk transition, rather than pressing into her feet and leaning back against the reins. And Sprinx will learn to listen to Leslie's center and come to walk in better balance, rather than propping against her front legs. The resulting walk will have better energy, and Leslie and Sprinx will stay in balance and harmony.

Exercises for Leslie: *Bounce in Rhythm 1–4; Abdominal Curls; Crisscross; Plank on Mat: Knees and Feet; Plank on Ball; Leg Lifts on Ball.*

Some people advise you to sit *heavily* on the seat bone in the direction of travel to accomplish lateral work. I fear this can disrupt balance in both you and your horse. A dramatic shift in your weight can cause your horse to fall, rather than to carry himself, in the direction of travel. This advice also risks your twisting out of correct alignment. I suggest that you sit *to* the direction of travel, keeping your pelvis level. For example, if you are doing a leg-yield to the right, sit to the right as if you are creating a tiny space that will allow your horse room to move to the right underneath you. This allows you to stay balanced, align your shoulders over your pelvis, and shift toward the direction of travel. By keeping your pelvis level and balanced (not heavily weighted on one side), you preserve body alignment and are more likely to have equal access to both rein and legs aids to precisely direct your horse's energy. In the energy diagram with *up* and *out* arrows, add an arrow directing the horse to the side, and send your energy along that line (see fig. 5.20, p. 194).

RIDING EXERCISE to Improve Timing of Aids

The leg-yield is a great exercise to practice working with your horse's gaits and applying aids at a logical time to improve your horse's response. It helps you and your horse move together. The example below describes the aids of a leg-yield to the left, with your horse moving away from your right leg. I'll describe doing the leg-yield from the quarterline of the arena to the arena wall.

1 Turn down the quarterline on the right rein. Establish a straight line with an active trot.

2 Feel the right-left stepping of your horse's hind legs.

3 When the right leg steps under, add extra movement or swing of your right leg to direct the right hind leg to cross in front of the left hind leg.

4 Keep your left rein supporting so your horse doesn't fall out the left shoulder.

5 Be sure to keep a ground-covering trot during the exercise, with your mental metronome ticking away, "right-left-right-left."

6 During the lateral movement, however, change the words for the mental metronome to "over" (for the right hind leg) and "forward" (for the left hind leg): "over-forward-over-forward." In this way, impulsion is maintained, and the lateral aid from your right leg occurs when your horse can respond (right hind leg in the air).

7 Sit in the direction of travel without leaning or twisting. In this leg-yield to the left, imagine your torso, balanced and aligned, going both forward and a bit to the left, as if making room, or a space, underneath the left side of your body for your horse to move into (fig. 5.21).

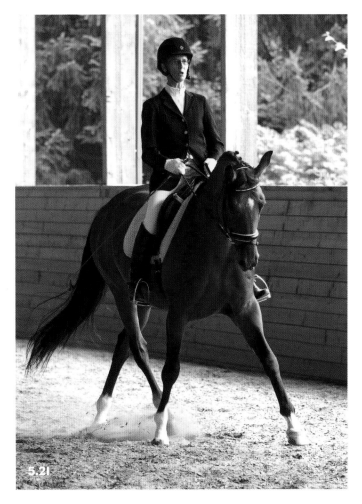

5.21

I ride DG in a leg-yield to the left, working to give logically timed aids while keeping my posture and spine alignment stable. I tend to be a "right-sided" rider, so it is easy for me to try and "help" DG go to the left by shifting my weight too much to the left. This risks her falling on her left shoulder, rather than carrying me left with her right hind leg, which she'd rather not do. Correct posture and balance, again, facilitate training. With vigilance of my body position, I can more readily perceive an evasion from her and correct it with consistency and tact. Further, correct balance allows me to stay in control of my leg aids; poor balance leads to leg-muscle tension. Useful exercises to solidify lateral balance: Pelvic Rocking on Ball: Side to Side; Side Planks on Mat: Knees; Side Planks on Mat: Feet.

Balanced Riding Is Efficient, Beautiful, and Healthy

There are many details to keep track of while riding, and it is easy to think only about what your horse is doing. You owe it to your horse to also consider *yourself*: to ask if your position and balance strategies are either causing or contributing to a training problem. And you owe it to yourself to keep track of yourself, and keep yourself from falling into unproductive and unhealthy postural and balance habits. With every step ask, "Where am I? Where is my body? Am I balanced? Am I moving with the gait?" After all, *you* are the cognitive member of the horse-rider pair, equipped with the analytical capabilities to solve problems. Be sure to include yourself as a potential part of a training problem, and use the Rider Fundamentals—Mental Focus, Proper Posture, Leg and Arm Control, and Understanding Movement—to assess your contribution to the problem and find solutions. As you develop these skills, you will be able to communicate with light aids and progress toward a wonderful state of balance and harmony with your horse. You will also be using your body in a way that minimizes strain so you can ride for years to come.

A Pretty Picture

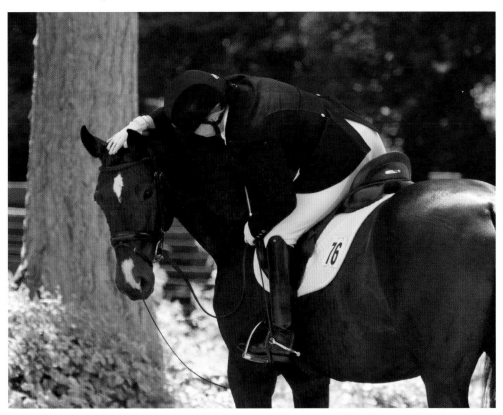

*Caryn Bujnowski gives Dylan a well-deserved pat. I often find myself telling riders to "give themselves"
a pat after a good ride. A successful ride is not random and won't happen without your commitment
to quality and attention to your position and function. Use the Rider Fundamentals to keep yourself
on track every step of the ride with Mental Focus, Proper Posture, Body Control—Legs and Arms, and
Understanding Movement. Enjoy the challenge!*

Learn More!

You can discover more ways to keep your riding body healthy and beautifully balanced for years to come by visiting my website: **www.riderpilates.com.**

RiderPilates® LLC
19610 NE 116th Street
Redmond, WA 98053
Cell: 425.246.9033

Complete List of Rider Fundamental Exercises

Suggested Workouts

Here are a few easy-to-follow and effective workout routines from exercises in this book.

Pre-Ride Warm-Up

Before you ride, take about 10 minutes to organize your body with this sequence of exercises. These movements can be done on a chair or a bale of hay instead of a ball, so you can do them in your barn before you ride. This sequence is designed to remind you of your body tools to improve your balance, awareness, and function before you get in the saddle.

1 Rib Cage Breathing 2 (use your hands on your torso rather than a stretchy band)—p. 15

2 Pelvic Rocking on Ball: Front to Back—p. 35

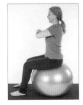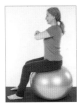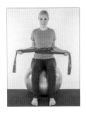

3 Pelvic Rocking on Ball: Side to Side—p. 69

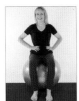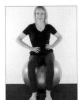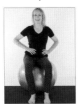

4 Spine Stretch Forward, alternating with Spine Extension: Scarecrow—pp. 39 & 41

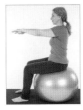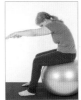
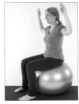

5 Spine Twist on Ball—p. 70

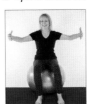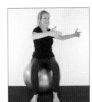

6 *Hug-a-Tree: Both Arms—p. 135*

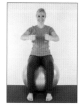 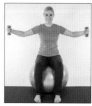

7 *Hug-a-Tree: Single Arm—p. 136*

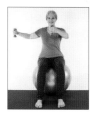 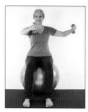

8 *Chest Expansion—p. 137*

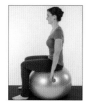 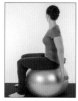

9 *Leg Lifts on Ball—p. 118*

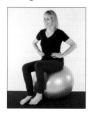

10 *Deep Rotator, Piriformis Stretch: Sitting—p. 99*

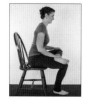

11 *Hamstring Stretch: Standing—p. 98*

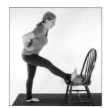

Basic Workout

Here are the basic versions of the exercises described in this book. With this workout you will develop the skills and body tools described in the Rider Fundamentals: *Mental Focus, Proper Posture, Leg and Arm Control,* and *Understanding Movement.* Plus, the beginning bouncing sequence hones your ability to maintain a steady tempo and warms up your body.

On-the-Ball Warm-Up

1 *Bounce in Rhythm 1—p. 21*

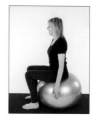 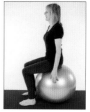

2 *Bounce in Rhythm 2: Arm Swings—p. 160*

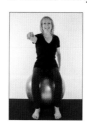

3 *Bounce in Rhythm 4: Ball Jacks—p. 161*

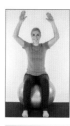 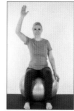 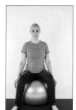 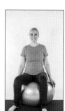

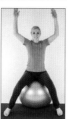 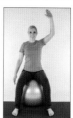 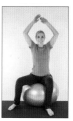 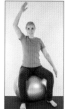

On-the-Ball Spine Awareness Warm-Up

4 Rib Cage Breathing 2—p. 15

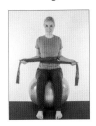

5 Pelvic Rocking on Ball: Front to Back—p. 35

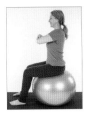 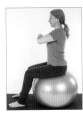 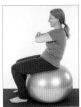

6 Pelvic Rocking on Ball: Side to Side—p. 69

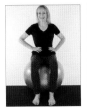 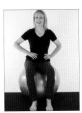 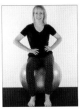

7 Spine Stretch Forward, alternating with
Spine Extension: Scarecrow—pp. 39 & 41

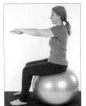 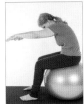
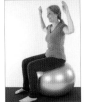

8 Spine Twist on Ball—p. 70

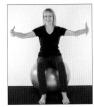 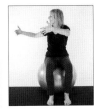 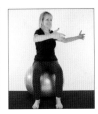

On-the-Mat Core Work

9 Abdominal Curls—p. 36

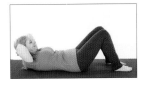 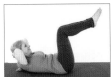

10 Crisscross—p. 44

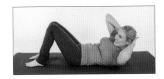

11 Spine Extension on Mat—p. 37

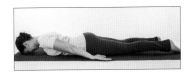

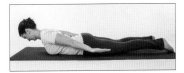

12 Back Stretch—p. 38

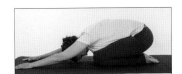

13 *Plank on Mat: Knees—p. 48*

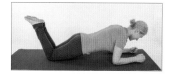

14 *Side Plank on Mat: Knees—p. 71*

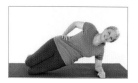

15 *Quadruped: Single—p. 51*

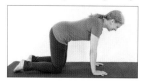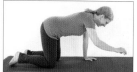

On-the-Mat Leg Work

16 *Knee Circles—p. 114*

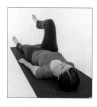

17 *Pelvic Bridge: Simple—p. 92*

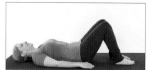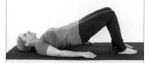

18 *Pelvic Bridge: Single Leg—p. 93*

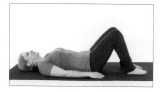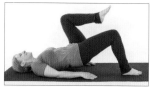

19 *Deep Rotator, Piriformis Stretch—p. 99*

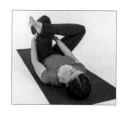

20 *Ball Tongs: Squeezes (on right)—p. 102*

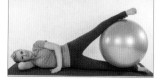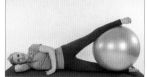

21 *Straight Legs—p. 107*

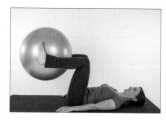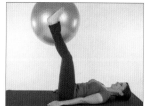

22 *Ball Tongs: Squeezes (on left)—p. 102*

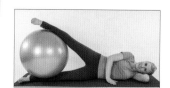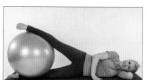

On-the-Ball Arm Work

23 Hug-a-Tree: Both Arms—p. 135

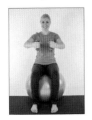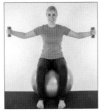

24 Chest Expansion—p. 137

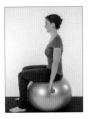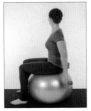

25 Shoulder Stretch—p. 143

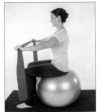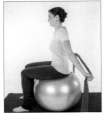

On-the-Mat Leg Stretches

26 Hip Flexor Stretch—p. 112

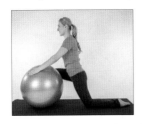

27 Hamstring Stretch (right)—p. 97

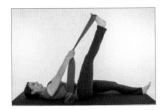

28 Abductor Stretch (right)—p. 105

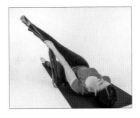

29 Hamstring Stretch (left)—p. 197

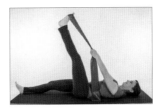

30 Abductor Stretch (left)—p. 105

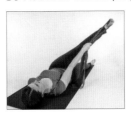

31 Adductor Stretch—p. 104

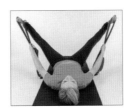

Intermediate Workout

This sequence of exercises is the more challenging version of the exercises described in this book. The workout further develops the skills and body tools of *Mental Focus, Proper Posture, Leg and Arm Control,* and *Understanding Movement.* Remember, when you are fatigued, you risk losing form, precision, and balance. It is better to keep great alignment and focus than to struggle with an exercise.

On-the-Ball Warm-Up

1 Bounce in Rhythm 1—p. 21

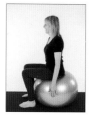
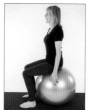

2 Bounce in Rhythm 2: Arm Swings—p. 160

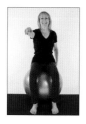

3 Bounce in Rhythm 3: Toe Tapping—p. 160

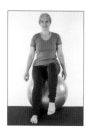

4 Bounce in Rhythm 4: Ball Jacks (including Single Arm and Single Leg variations)—p. 161

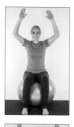
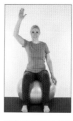
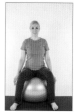
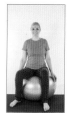

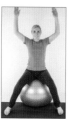
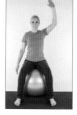
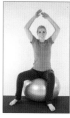
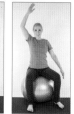

On-the-Ball Spine Awareness Warm-Up

5 Rib Cage Breathing 2—p. 15

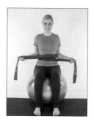

6 Pelvic Rocking on Ball: Front to Back—p. 35

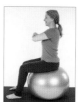
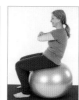
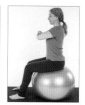

7 Pelvic Rocking on Ball: Side to Side—p. 69

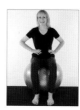
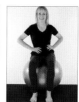
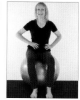

8 Spine Stretch Forward, alternating with Spine Extension: Scarecrow—pp. 39 & 41

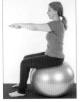
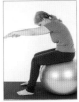

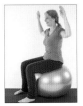
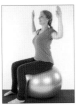

9 Spine Twist on Ball—p. 70

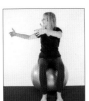
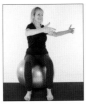

On-the-Mat Core Work

10 Abdominal Curls Sustained—p. 43

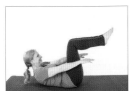
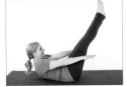

11 Crisscross Sustained—p. 44

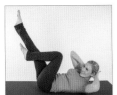
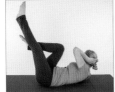

12 Spine Extension on Mat—p. 37

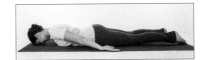

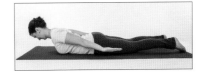

13 Back Stretch—p. 38

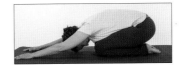

14 Plank on Mat: Feet—p. 49

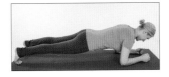

15 Side Plank on Mat: Feet—p. 72

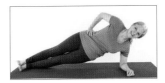

16 Quadruped: Diagonal—p. 52

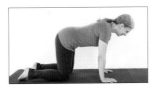
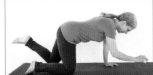

On-the-Mat Leg Work

17 Leg Circles—p. 115

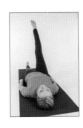
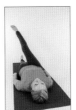
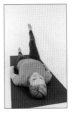
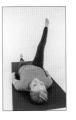

18 *Pelvic Bridge with Ball—p. 94*

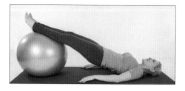

19 *Pelvic Bridge with Ball: Balance—p. 95*

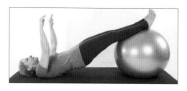

20 *Pelvic Bridge with Ball: Single Leg—p. 96*

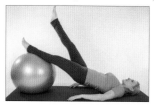

21 *Deep Rotator, Piriformis Stretch—p. 99*

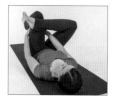

22 *Ball Tongs: Squeezes (on right without supporting left hand)—p. 102*

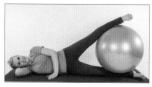 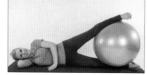

23 *Ball Tongs: Lifts (on right)—p. 103*

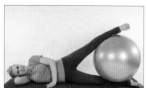 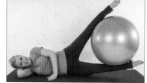

24 *Straight Legs—p. 107*

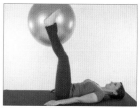 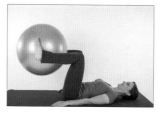

25 *Ball Tongs: Squeezes (on left without supporting right hand)—p. 102*

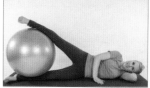 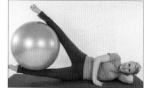

26 *Ball Tongs: Lifts (on left)—p. 103*

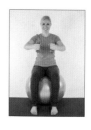 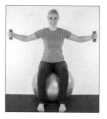

On-the-Ball Arm Work

27 *Hug-a-Tree: Both Arms—p. 135*

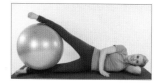 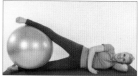

28 *Hug-a-Tree: Single Arm—p. 136*

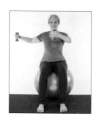 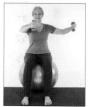

29 Chest Expansion—p. 137

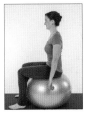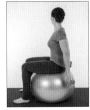

30 Shoulder Stretch—p. 143

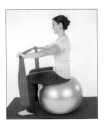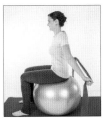

On-the-Mat Leg Stretches

31 Hip Flexor Stretch—p. 112

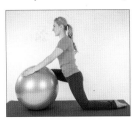

32 Hamstring Stretch (right)—p. 97

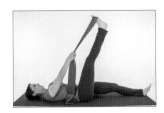

33 Abductor Stretch (right)—p. 105

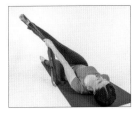

34 Hamstring Stretch (left)—p. 97

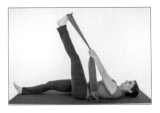

35 Abductor Stretch (left)—p. 105

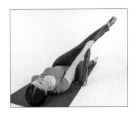

36 Adductor Stretch—p. 104

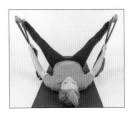

Bibliography

Bruckner, Peter and Khan, Karim. *Clinical Sports Medicine.* Australia: McGraw Hill, 2008.

Calais-Germain, Blandine. *Anatomy of Movement.* Seattle: Eastland Press, 1993.

Craig, Colleen. *Pilates on the Ball: The World's Most Popular Workout Using the Exercise Ball.* Rochester, VT: Healing Arts Press, 2001.

Craig, Colleen. *Strength Training on the Ball: A Pilates Approach to Optimal Strength and Balance.* Rochester, VT: Healing Arts Press, 2005.

Crawford, Elizabeth. *Balance on the Ball: Exercises Inspired by the Teachings of Joseph Pilates.* San Francisco: Equilibrio, 2000.

Jenkins, David B. *Hollinshead's Functional Anatomy of the Limbs and Back.* 7th ed. Philadelphia: W.B. Saunders Company, 1998.

Lessen, Deborah, editor. *The PMA Pilates Certification Exam Study Guide.* Miami: Pilates Method Alliance, 2005.

Pilates, Joseph H. Your Health: *A Corrective System of Exercising that Revolutionizes the Entire Field of Physical Education.* 1934. Reprint, Incline Village, NV: Presentation Dynamics, Inc., 1998.

Pilates, Joseph H. Pilates, and William J. Miller. *Pilates' Return to Life Through Contrology.* 1945. Reprint, Incline Village, NV: Presentation Dynamics, Inc., 1998.

Richardson, Carolyn, et al. *Therapeutic Exercise for Spinal Segmental Stabilization in Low Back Pain: Scientific Basis and Clinical Approach.* London: Churchill Livingstone, 1999.

Index

Page numbers in *italics* indicate illustrations.

Index